Insider's Guide to Gum Disease, Orthodontics and Dentistry

✦

What is not taught in dental school

Insider's Guide to Gum Disease, Orthodontics and Dentistry

✦

What is not taught in dental school

David C. DiBenedetto, D.M.D.

iUniverse, Inc.
New York Lincoln Shanghai

Insider's Guide to Gum Disease, Orthodontics and Dentistry
What is not taught in dental school

iUniverse books may be ordered through booksellers or by contacting:

iUniverse
2021 Pine Lake Road, Suite 100
Lincoln, NE 68512
www.iuniverse.com
1-800-Authors (1-800-288-4677)

Because of the dynamic nature of the Internet, any Web addresses or links contained in this book may have changed since publication and may no longer be valid.

The information, ideas, and suggestions in this book are not intended as a substitute for professional medical advice. Before following any suggestions contained in this book, you should consult your personal physician. Neither the author nor the publisher shall be liable or responsible for any loss or damage allegedly arising as a consequence of your use or application of any information or suggestions in this book.

ISBN: 978-0-595-48083-8 (pbk)
ISBN: 978-0-595-71680-7 (cloth)
ISBN: 978-0-595-60182-0 (ebk)

Printed in the United States of America

To my family

"The doctors are in the dark." Lorenzo's Oil.

I would like to thank my wife, Martha Moss, M.D., and my cousin Nancy DiBenedetto.

Contents

Preface

I want to present an insider's view of dentistry, a view encompassing the inside information that public relation brochures do not provide. Much dentistry today is performed for cosmetic reasons, for convenience, or for medical and legal reasons. Much such treatment is based largely on dogma. As dentists, we often forget that we are practitioners of a medical science and that the principles of medicine should apply to dentistry. Dentistry lacks good diagnostic, epidemiological, and research-based science

After reading my book, you will understand the importance of good occlusion, how orthodontists have failed us, and the many shortfalls of periodontics.

Occlusion is the study of how our teeth meet when our jaws come together. Occlusion is dynamic rather than static. Although occlusion is of crucial importance to dental health, very little is taught about it in dental school. Dentists have to learn it on their own.

The field of orthodontics is about aesthetics and does not concern itself on how our jaws function. Orthodontists claim that straightening teeth makes it easier to remove dental plaque and therefore makes teeth and gums healthier. However, multiple studies show that orthodontic treatment does not increase patients' chances of keeping their teeth later in life.

Millions of dollars each year are spent on diagnosis and treatment of periodontal disease. We are led to believe that most of us will eventually have it and lose our teeth from it. If periodontal disease is caused by a bacterial infection, why hasn't the incidence declined in the era of antibiotics? Appendicitis, tonsillitis, ulcers, Ludwig's angina, and leprosy have all declined. What treatment, then, works best for periodontal disease? More importantly, are we making any progress in controlling this disease?

Lastly, as dentists, we can't forget the important role that overall health plays in determining our dental health. Our teeth are held in our mouths by surrounding bone, and bone is a living tissue, part of a living body.

David C. DiBenedetto, D.M.D.

1

How Periodontists Think

The American Academy of Periodontology believes that periodontal diseases, including gingivitis and periodontitis, are serious infections that can lead to tooth loss if not treated quickly. According to the Academy, "Periodontal disease is a chronic bacterial infection that affects the gums and bone supporting the teeth." It can affect one tooth or many teeth and begins when the gums become inflamed because of the bacteria in plaque.

In gingivitis, which is the mildest form of the disease, the gums get red, swell, and bleed easily. Periodontists claim that gingivitis can lead to periodontitis, which is inflammation of the gums and other structures that support the teeth. It is believed that with time, plaque can spread and grow below the gum line. Then toxins produced by the bacteria in plaque irritate the gums, causing the body to turn on itself, breaking down the tissues and bone that support the teeth. This process causes the gums to separate from the teeth, forming spaces between the teeth and gums, called "pockets," which become infected. The pockets deepen as the disease progresses and more bone is destroyed. Finally the teeth become loose and have to be removed. Bone loss causes teeth to fall out.

If you are diagnosed with periodontal disease, your periodontist will most likely recommend surgery. Millions of dollars are spent every year to treat bone loss. The dental community doesn't understand that there are many other causes of bone loss. What factors, then, are responsible for bone loss?

One notable one is occlusion, the contact between the teeth when the jaw is in its various positions. Occlusal forces cause teeth to wear and to become loose. Another is poor health. Unhealthy hosts include smokers, patients with undiagnosed diseases such as osteoporosis and diabetes, sufferers of vitamin deficiencies, and other patients who have poor nutrition. Occlusal forces may also be responsible for other medical conditions such as migraines, temporomandibular joint (TMJ) disorder, and bruxism.

Patients seek dental help for damaged teeth on a regular basis, but dentists rarely diagnose the true problem. So, although they treat the damage to teeth or gums and bone caused by occlusal forces, they usually identify its cause as something else, such as periodontal disease or brushing too hard. Sometimes they may not even attempt to identify a cause.

Dentists always talk about prevention—brush your teeth, use mouth rinses, and floss to prevent cavities and gingivitis. When it comes to occlusion, however, there is not enough talk about preventing occlusal problems. After serious consequences have developed because of bad occlusal guidance or ignorance, then the talk turns to treatment. Why doesn't treatment come up earlier? Because there's no money in prevention! Most insurance companies will not pay for preventive advice and treatment either. Why wait until group guidance or balancing side guidance hurts the body before we treat it? Read further to understand what guidance is all about.

Most dentists do not pay attention to their patients' occlusion. They just treat a patient's immediate problem without taking occlusal factors into consideration. They don't seem to understand or care about the consequences to their patients' teeth and overall health due to poor occlusion. Part of the reason is that dentists don't learn about occlusion in dental school. Dentists are just taught how to fill and drill or cut and sew.

But dentists need to be more concerned about occlusion so they can help their patients maintain their occlusal health and fix any problems with their occlusion so they won't be in pain when they chew, as well as to stop bone loss and to prevent headaches, among other symptoms.

2

Balance, Wear and Tear, and Symmetry

Balance, wear and tear, and symmetry are paramount, long-term factors.

This assumption leads to the important question: "How do the jaws work?" Let's think about balance, first in terms of our car tires and then in terms of our jaws.

The definition of balance is the uniform distribution of mass about an axis of rotation, where the center of gravity is in the same location as the center of rotation. This means a tire, mounted on the wheel and the axle of the car, is in balance when the mass of the tire is uniformly distributed around the axle.

Maintaining the equal balance of your tires is critical to saving wear and tear on them as well as ensuring that your vehicle performs optimally. Balanced tires are critical to performance and safety when your car turns or deviates from a straight line. Balanced tires can mean the difference between a good or a bad driving experience. A tire that is out of balance can adversely affect ride quality; such imbalance can also shorten the life of your tires, bearings, shocks, and other parts of the suspension system.

Just as balanced tires are vital to a car's performance, our jaws also need to be balanced to maintain good dental health. The way teeth are

4

positioned in our jaws determines whether our jaws are balanced and how they are balanced.

The upper jaw is fixed to our skull. The lower jaw has three primary movements plus combination of movements. It opens and closes, moves from side to side, and moves forward and backward. But the teeth positioned in the jaws limit the movements of the lower jaw. This limitation is very important. The lower jaw cannot touch the upper jaw because the teeth are in the way. So how does tooth position affect the movement of the lower jaw?

lower jaw movements

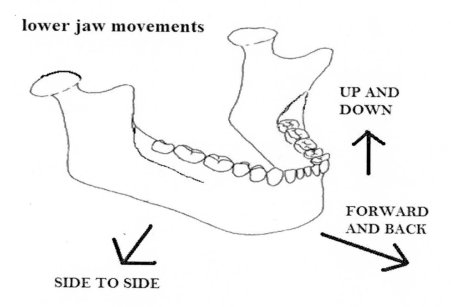

UP AND DOWN

FORWARD AND BACK

SIDE TO SIDE

The lower jaw is connected to two temporomandibular joints, or TMJs. That means this one bone, the lower jawbone, also called the mandible, is connected to two joints. These two temporomandibular joints, along with the muscles of the face, work together to move the lower jaw.

It is important to remember that the lower jaw cannot touch the upper jaw because the teeth are in the way. If the lower jaw moves forward and back and is closed, some teeth must touch. If the lower jaw moves right to left and then is closed, some teeth must touch. If the jaws are of normal size, we can then determine how the teeth are placed by what teeth touch when the closed lower jaw moves in different directions.

Centric occlusion is the position our teeth are in when we repeatedly close down on our back teeth (habitual position). Centric relation is when the head of the condyle of the lower jaw is positioned in the most superior anterior position of the TMJ, a very retruded or some dentists claim the most retruded and relaxed position for the lower jaw. Centric occlusion can never be more retruded than centric relation.

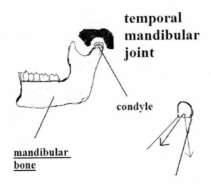

arrows represent the direction the head of the condlye can move in the tmj

In centric occlusion or centric relation, the back teeth should touch. The back teeth should touch in an up-and-down movement only. How should the front teeth touch in centric occlusion? Because the movement in centric occlusion is up-and-down, or opening and closing, the front teeth should not touch edge-to-edge. That's because edge-to-edge touching of the front teeth will cause increased wear or chipping. The ideal situation is when the lower front teeth touch the upper front teeth from behind in centric occlusion. In a good occlusion, when the lower jaw is shifted to one side or the other, the back teeth should not touch when the jaws are brought together. The front teeth prevent and protect the back teeth from touching. That's because the forces on the back teeth will change from an up-and-down movement to tipping or shearing. Tipping or shearing forces are detrimental. They cause eventual harm to teeth, jaws, muscles, and joints.

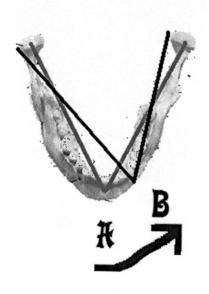

WHEN THE LOWER JAW MOVES LATERALLY, FROM A TO B, AND THE JAW IS CLOSED SOME TEETH MUST TOUCH. THE LOWER JAW CAUSES TWISTING FORCES AGAINST THE UPPER TEETH

ANTERIOR GUIDANCE VS GROUP

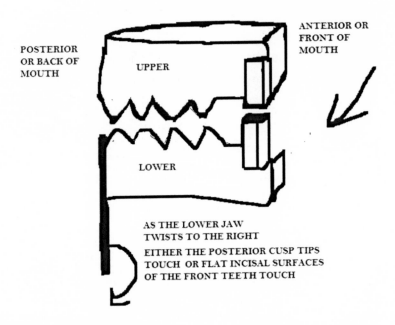

POSTERIOR
OR BACK OF
MOUTH

UPPER

ANTERIOR OR
FRONT OF
MOUTH

LOWER

AS THE LOWER JAW
TWISTS TO THE RIGHT
EITHER THE POSTERIOR CUSP TIPS
TOUCH OR FLAT INCISAL SURFACES
OF THE FRONT TEETH TOUCH

Now let's talk about occlusal guidance. Guidance is the term used for the teeth that touch in lateral excursions. The upper canine teeth are the strongest teeth in the mouth. They are the longest teeth, and they have the greatest amount of hard tooth structure surrounding the nerve. They are positioned at the pivot points in the jaws. The canines can withstand tipping forces better than any other tooth because of their location and strength. Canine guidance occurs when the lower jaw moves away from centric occlusion and the canines become the only teeth that touch when the jaws come together. **In other words, when the lower jaw moves to the right or to the left and then comes together, the canines are the only teeth that touch.**

In anterior guidance, any of the upper four incisors are the only teeth that touch when the lower jaw is moved from centric to side-to-side, and the jaws are together. So in anterior guidance, the teeth in between the canines, the incisor teeth rather than the canines, will touch when the jaw moves from side to side.

In group guidance (or, as it is more commonly known, group function), all the pressure during the lateral movement of the jaw is progressively borne by the back teeth. In any movement away from centric, the lower back teeth will hit the upper back teeth on the side of that movement. So if you move your lower jaw to the right, keeping your teeth together, the lower right back teeth will touch the upper right back teeth.

POSTERIOR TEETH

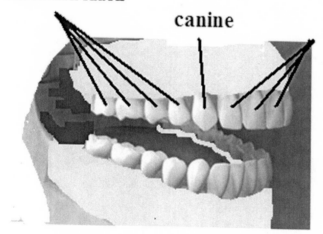

Balancing side guidance (or balancing side interference) happens when you move your jaw to one side and your back teeth hit the teeth on the opposite side. That means that if you move your lower jaw to the right, the lower back teeth on the left side will hit the upper left back teeth. This causes unnatural and harmful lateral forces on these back teeth, forces that can cause damage to bone and/or pain in the teeth and/or the joints.

balancing side guidance

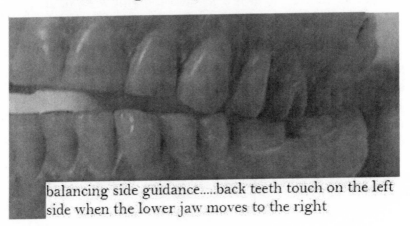

balancing side guidance.....back teeth touch on the left side when the lower jaw moves to the right

notice the open bite between the front teeth

Protrusive interference occurs when you move your lower jaw forward from centric, bringing the teeth together, and the back teeth touch.

Our teeth wear out just like our knees, hips, and backs. Tipping, and shearing forces are like twisting forces. We all are aware that twisting forces hurt the knees, hips, and back.

Ultimately *all occlusions will wear out*. The best engineering to slow down wear and tear on our teeth, the bone around our teeth, and the joints that move our lower jaw is canine guidance.

CANINE GUIDANCE

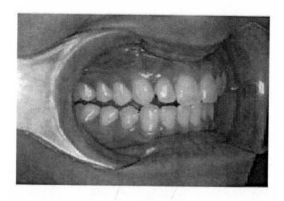

NOTICE THE SPACE BETWEEN THE POSTERIOR TEETH AS THE LOWER JAW MOVES TO THE RIGHT WHILE THE JAWS ARE BROUGHT TOGETHER

Canine guidance, also called cuspid-protected occlusion, improves the longevity of the teeth and our jaws. Over time, the canines will wear down from this occlusion, and this wear can be manifested by gingival recession (bone loss on the facial surface), which causes the root of the canine tooth to be exposed. This gingival recession often causes tooth sensitivity. I believe more gingival recession occurs from normal wear and tear than from brushing too hard or from periodontal disease.

After recession comes abfraction. Over time, the tipping forces on the teeth can cause abfraction. Abfraction appears as a notch or cavity on the facial surface of the tooth near or under the gum. It occurs where the gum has receded. Most often the notch can be sharp. Although using a toothbrush with hard bristles and not brushing properly can cause the loss of tooth structure at the gum line, this is not abfraction. Abfraction usually occurs after gingival recession. The same tipping and torqueing forces are responsible for both gingival recession and abfraction.

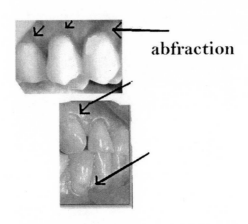

abfraction

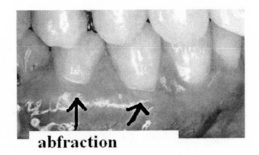

abfraction

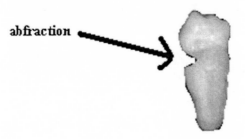

abfraction

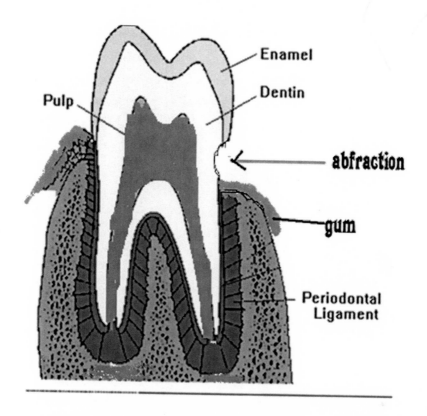

We do not have good animal models demonstrating abfraction lesions, but old cats develop FORLs—feline odontoclastic resorptive lesions. We do not know what causes FORL formation, but we think it is abfraction. We know FORL cannot be caused from brushing too hard because cats do not brush their teeth.

In anterior guidance, abfraction will occur on the anterior teeth. So gum recession can occur on the anterior teeth when a patient has anterior guidance. As I mentioned before, anterior guidance can also cause the front teeth to chip.

When the lower back teeth hit the upper back teeth at tipping angles, many unpleasant things will happen. Teeth will break; teeth will move; teeth will have mobility; teeth will rotate; gums will recede.

There will be abfraction on the back teeth, there will be misdiagnoses, and there will be pain in some teeth, leading to root canal treatment. There will be bone loss around back teeth; crowns will fall off; dental implants will fail; bruxism or teeth grinding may occur; headaches and muscles spasms will occur in some people; and tooth decay will occur in unusual places. Increased stress, these tipping and twisting forces, will also make the tooth more prone to decay.

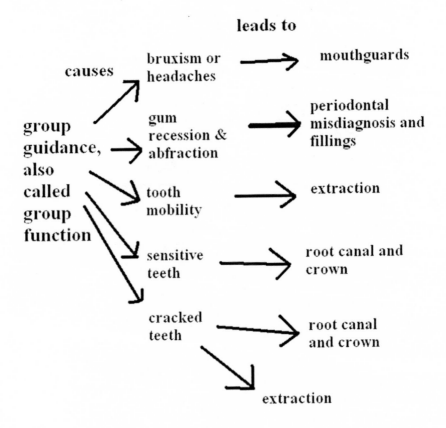

Group guidance, therefore, causes many problems. It seems that the patients who suffer from bruxism are less likely to get abfraction or tooth mobility. It's amazing that patients who experience bruxism or headaches because of group guidance will get almost instant relief when they are taken out of group guidance and put into anterior or canine guidance. The effect is similar to how a car rides better when the wheels are balanced and aligned. The car doesn't shake with good alignment.

We don't know why patients experience instant relief. But the more important question is, "How long will someone endure group guidance before we see these problems manifest?" That time will depend on how much chewing or talking the patient does, or how often the patient uses his or her jaws. However, not all cases of TMJ, bruxism, or headaches are caused by group guidance or balancing side guidance. We need more comprehensive knowledge, including epidemiology, to know how many incidences of these problems are due to guidance anomalies.

Many times, when patients are relieved of group guidance and put into anterior guidance, their teeth meet better, feel better, and chew better. Some patients who have come into my office with group guidance have told me that they want me to remove all their back teeth because of the pain. I believe many root canals that are performed today on these back teeth could have been prevented if the patient did not experience group guidance. Many times dentists perform root canals on back teeth because the patients have vague pain in those teeth. This pain may be the result of hairline fractures caused by the tipping forces of group or balancing-side guidance. Root canal treatments done on these teeth are not as successful as those performed on teeth that have been insulted by decay.

Teeth break more often under group guidance, and that means more crowns are needed on those teeth. Here's a really important fact about group guidance—it causes gum recession on the back teeth. Unfortunately, many dentists confuse this gum recession with periodontal disease, which may lead to unnecessary treatment for periodontal disease. Periodontal treatment under these circumstances does not address the etiology of the problem.

Balancing side guidance, or balancing side interference, as discussed earlier, occurs on the opposite side of group function. Balancing side guidance, which may occur at the same time as group guidance, is probably worse than group guidance. Having balancing side function at the same time as having group guidance may limit the effects of the two or compound the problem. There are different degrees of balancing side function, which is not measured by any means I know. Some people who have balancing side function may be able to put their fingers (maybe ten to fifteen millimeters of space) between the front teeth when the jaws are closed in excursion. For others, the space between the front teeth may only be one or two millimeters. Balancing side guidance will make a person appear to have an open bite between the teeth when shifting the jaw.

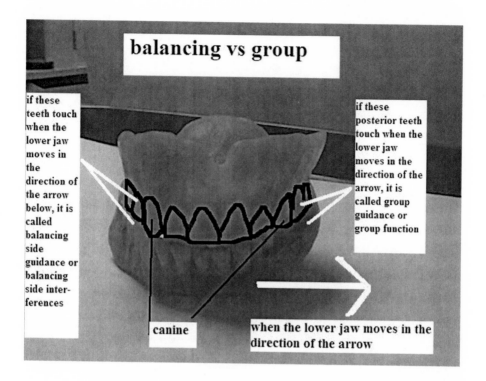

balancing vs group

if these teeth touch when the lower jaw moves in the direction of the arrow below, it is called balancing side guidance or balancing side inter-ferences

if these posterior teeth touch when the lower jaw moves in the direction of the arrow, it is called group guidance or group function

canine

when the lower jaw moves in the direction of the arrow

Very often wisdom teeth that have erupted will cause the balancing side guidance. Occlusion might have been fine until the wisdom teeth erupted.

Some patients may have anterior guidance or canine guidance on one side and group guidance on the other side.

3

Occlusion

The orthodontic view of occlusion is that almost everyone has a malocclusion, or bad bite. Malocclusion most often occurs when there is too much room or not enough room in the jaw (or jaws) for the teeth. Malocclusion is crooked teeth. No one has an ideal occlusion. Almost everyone needs braces. However, the opposing view says that there is no pathology associated with a malocclusion. Malocclusion is judged by appearance. Appearance is important in our society today. But satisfactory appearance that is not coupled with good guidance is detrimental to jaws, teeth, and face. Appearance is subjective, not objective. Appearance is not a functional factor.

Edward Hartley Angle, the father of modern orthodontics, created the classifications of malocclusion, based on the placement of the first molars. According to Angle, malocclusions are mainly divided into three types: Class I, Class II, and Class III.

In Class I malocclusion, the jaws are aligned properly, and the bite is satisfactory. The top teeth line up with the bottom teeth, but the teeth are crooked, crowded, or turned.

In Class II malocclusion, the upper and lower jaws don't line up properly, and the upper teeth protrude (stick out past the lower teeth). This is also called an overbite, or buck teeth.

In Class II, division II malocclusion, the upper incisors lean back. This position of the incisors generally gives anterior guidance.

In Class III skeletal malocclusion, the lower jaw protrudes, and the lower teeth stick out past the upper teeth. This is also called an underbite.

Malocclusion can range from mild to severe and can be skeletal or dental in origin. If one jaw is larger than the other, it is a skeletal malocclusion. If the jaws are of normal size, the condition is a dental malocclusion. It is hard to correct a skeletal malocclusion with braces alone.

Orthodontists like Angle are not interested in canine guidance or anterior guidance per se; they are concerned with how the teeth look. They want their patients to have attractive smiles. A pretty smile includes a nice profile of the upper lip and no rotations of teeth. They also want the midline of the teeth to correspond with the midline of the face.

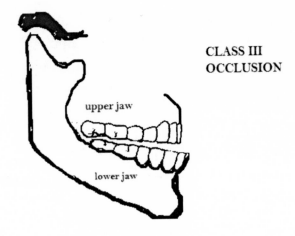

CLASS III
OCCLUSION

upper jaw

lower jaw

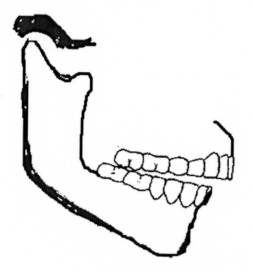

class II bite..... notice
that the front teeth
protrude

4

Sleep Apnea

How about centric and the hinge position?

Some occlusion "masters" feel centric occlusion should equal centric relation. This is a very retruded position. These "masters" feel centric relation is the most relaxed position for the TMJ. They most often construct the teeth so this will occur. But this position has an undesirable consequence, and it is sleep apnea.

Retruding the mandible may cause sleep apnea, a medical condition in which a person may briefly stop breathing while sleeping. There are several types of sleep apnea. In obstructive sleep apnea, which is caused by a blockage of the airway, the soft tissue in the back of the throat collapses and closes the airway during sleep. In central sleep apnea, the brain fails to signal the muscles to breathe. In mixed apnea, both those conditions occur. When sleep apnea occurs, the brain briefly wakes people up so they can start breathing again. But that means their sleep is constantly disrupted, so they are always tired.

Left untreated, sleep apnea can cause high blood pressure and other cardiovascular diseases, memory problems, weight gain, impotency, and headaches. In addition, people who suffer from sleep apnea are often unable to perform at work and may cause car accidents because of the dysfunction caused by their lack of good sleep.

Many patients with obstructive sleep apnea have thick necks and lower-face abnormalities, which may include a small chin, small upper jaw, and small mandible. One current treatment for sleep apnea involves using a dental device to make the mandible protrude while the person is sleeping. Protruding the lower jaw opens the airway. Retruding the mandible, on the other hand, may cause the airway to get smaller. In CPR, doctors or medical technicians bring the lower jaw forward to create a good airway. Any action that makes an already restricted airway smaller is undesirable.

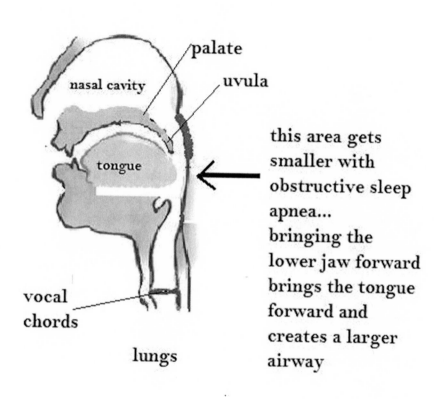

this area gets smaller with obstructive sleep apnea...
bringing the lower jaw forward brings the tongue forward and creates a larger airway

5

Epidemiology

Epidemiology is the "study of the distribution and frequency of disease or injury in human populations and the factors that make groups susceptible to disease or injury." Epidemiology stresses the health of groups or populations. From epidemiology we learn how much disease is present, the causes of the disease, and how well it is controlled.

Specifically, the best epidemiology that we have in dentistry concerns tooth decay, especially in children. We know what public health measures help in fighting tooth decay—fluorides and sealants. New epidemiology from insurance companies has shown that sealants are cost-effective in reducing new decay.

But we lack good epidemiology when it comes to periodontal disease, orthodontic malocclusion, TMJ pain, tooth loss, bone loss, inflammation, and guidance of occlusion.

Let's look at tooth loss, for example. What causes it? When does a dentist determine that a tooth must be extracted? When should a tooth be removed? There are a number of reasons that your dentist might recommend that you have a tooth, or even several teeth, extracted. Here are some of these reasons.

1. Wisdom teeth. Much controversy surrounds the issue of whether and when wisdom teeth should be extracted. The rationale behind the extraction of the wisdom teeth is that most people don't have enough room in their mouths for these third molars. When the wisdom teeth erupt, they change guidance. If they don't fully erupt and remain partially impacted, they can cause pain and possibly infection. Should impacted wisdom teeth that aren't causing problems be left alone, since the removal of deeply impacted teeth can damage surrounding nerves? Many dentists often call removal of wisdom teeth a preventive tactic.

2. To create room for orthodontic treatment (braces) to fix crooked or crowded teeth. If there is a serious lack of space for teeth, and all the teeth can't fit in the jaw, dentists will pull some in preparation for braces. That is because the dentist is trying to align the patient's teeth but can only do so within the confines of the size of the patient's jaws.

3. Trauma. Cracked teeth may need to be removed and avulsed teeth cannot always be reimplanted. Do all cracked teeth have to be removed? Well, that depends on the nature of the crack. The only part of a cracked tooth that can be predictably repaired is the part that's above the bone.

4. Root canal treatment is needed, but the patient doesn't want a root canal. Root canal therapy, also known as endodontic therapy, is a dental treatment designed to repair teeth with infected or damaged pulp. Because the pulp provides blood and nutrients to the tooth, damage to the pulp is serious and can result in the death of a tooth. Root canal therapy is recommended when damage to the tooth's pulp becomes visible or when the tooth is dead. Although dentists recommend root canal therapy to save the tooth, many patients would rather have the tooth extracted. In addition, teeth that are unsuitable candidates for root canal treatment should be extracted.

5. Root canal treatment has failed. If, after root canal treatment, there is still necrotic tissue present in the root canal system, then the treatment has failed, and the tooth may need to be removed if a second root canal treatment or surgery is not performed. Signs of failed root canal treatment can include mild to severe tooth pain and tenderness or swelling in the gums surrounding the tooth.

6. Dentures or aesthetics. If the patient already has missing teeth, then an easy and quick alternative is to remove the remaining teeth and put dentures in. Unfortunately, many patients opt for this treatment.

7. Implants. In some cases, it may be easier to remove the tooth and put in an implant than to restore the tooth. A dental implant is an artificial tooth root that is placed into a patient's jaw to hold a replacement tooth or bridge. The most common implant used today is an endosteal, or in-the-bone, implant, which is screwed into the jawbone. Each implant can hold one or more prosthetic teeth.

8. Occlusion. Because the tooth has taken so much force for so long, it has loosened up, and bone around it has been destroyed.

9. Too much decay. If the tooth cannot be restored, even with a root canal, because the decay is deep or because so much of its structure has been eaten away, then extraction is necessary.

10. Periodontal disease. Many dentists are led to believe that chronic destructive periodontal disease is responsible for more loss of teeth than cavities, particularly in older people. This is why further study of epidemiology is needed. We are perpetuating a myth and deluding ourselves when we say most adult teeth are lost to periodontal disease.

11. Patients' wishes. It is very hard to determine when teeth are extracted or removed for ease of treatment. It may be easier for the patient, in regard to time, comfort, aesthetics, or money, to have teeth removed and either have implants placed or dentures inserted.

Bone and bone loss Our teeth are held in our mouths by a ligament that goes from the root of the tooth to the bone surrounding the tooth. A ligament is connective tissue that holds two bones together or holds a tooth to the jawbone. The roots of our teeth are hidden, but once our gums start to recede, the roots of the teeth become visible. When baby teeth fall out, we don't see any root. That is because the root dissolves before the adult tooth erupts. We don't know why the root resorbs on baby teeth without affecting the nearby adult teeth. We also don't know why the upper baby canines are usually the last teeth to fall out among the primary teeth. Is it because the upper (maxillary) canines, the most important teeth in our mouths, need added time to develop?

The transition from primary dentition stage to adult dentition begins with the loss of the baby incisors at about six years old. Because the upper canines erupt last, this mixed dentition stage still needs good guidance. The incisors that erupt have mamelons—projections on the top of the teeth. Other teeth do not have mamelons. These mamelons wear down after a few years. Since chipping and wear can occur from anterior guidance, mamelons could be a protective mechanism for the dentition until the canines erupt.

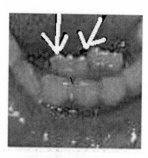

mamelons

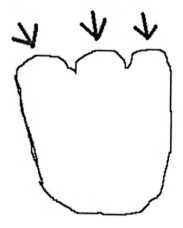

On average, the roots of the upper anterior teeth are twice the length of the crown, with the longest in the upper canine teeth. The anterior teeth consist of two canines and four incisors. The posterior or back teeth consist of all teeth behind the canines. The back teeth have the shortest roots; the roots of the anterior teeth are the longest. Because anterior teeth have longer roots than back teeth, they handle guidance of the jaws better.

As the gums recede, we lose both the bone around the tooth and the ligament that goes from the tooth to the bone. This is called the periodontal ligament, commonly abbreviated as the PDL. It is a group of specialized connective tissue fibers that attach a tooth to the bone within which it sits. The PDL helps the teeth withstand the compressive forces that occur during chewing. The PDL acts like a shock absorber for the tooth, much like the shock absorber in a car. The PDL and the bone around the teeth hold the teeth in the jawbone.

Bone loss can occur from the forces that cause abfraction. The location of the bone loss is determined by guidance—group guidance, anterior guidance, canine guidance, protrusive interference, and balancing side guidance—in other words, the workings of the jaw. How the jaw works determines where the bone loss will occur.

Bone loss can occur on the teeth adjacent to the space left from an extracted tooth. Bone loss can occur from brushing the gums too hard. Bone loss can occur from the decay that goes under the gums. Bone loss can occur from orthodontic movement. Bone loss can occur from a tooth that doesn't erupt properly. Bone loss can occur when a tooth over erupts because the opposing tooth is missing.

However, most periodontists strongly believe that the harmful bacteria that reside around the gums cause almost all bone loss. This bacteria produces inflammation, leading to bone loss around the teeth. Periodontists call this bone loss that comes from bacteria plaque periodontal disease.

The problem with this scenario is that periodontal disease does not satisfy **Koch's postulates**. On the other hand, tooth decay does satisfy Koch's postulates. In 1890, the German physician and bacteriologist Robert Koch published his criteria for judging whether a given bacteria is the cause of a given disease, bringing some much-needed scientific clarity to what was then a very confused and undefined field.

Koch was the first scientist to firmly establish the link between germs and disease. A doctor with a small rural practice in Germany, Koch had an interest in microscopic studies that led him eventually to identify the bacteria that cause the disease anthrax, which was then a common killer of sheep, cows and, occasionally, farmers. From there, Koch worked to develop the means by which he could prove without a doubt that these organisms were indeed to blame.

Koch's work on anthrax was published in 1876 and touched off a revolution within the medical community. By the turn of the century, scientists working primarily under the tutelage of Koch and Louis Pasteur had identified most major bacilli, including those responsible for anthrax, gonorrhea, pneumonia, typhoid fever, septicemia, tuberculosis, cholera, plague, tetanus, diphtheria, and meningitis.

Koch's postulates are as follows.

1. The bacteria must be present in every case of the disease.

2. The bacteria must be isolated from the host with the disease and grown in pure culture.

3. The specific disease must be reproduced when a pure culture of the bacteria is inoculated into a healthy susceptible host.

4. The bacteria must be recoverable from the experimentally infected host.

Bacteria and dental plaque that supposedly cause periodontal disease have never been isolated from the host, grown in a pure culture, or reproduced in another healthy host; they have never been recovered from that new infected host. Also, bacteria have never been isolated even from the diseased bone of a patient with "periodontal disease." Unbelievable!

But periodontists get around Koch's postulates by saying periodontal disease is an infection that is caused by many organisms, and because multiple organisms act differently from single organisms, they don't necessarily have to fit into Koch's postulates.

Periodontal disease is a disease that is measured from baseline. Baseline is a reference point that is used to indicate the initial condition against which future measurements are compared.

Dentists cannot diagnosis active disease. In many ways, it is similar to measuring osteoporosis. Periodontal disease is measuring bone level, and osteoporosis is measuring bone density at a given point in time. It doesn't tell you if things are getting better or worse—it is necessary to look at baseline and compare the two at two different intervals of time. I repeat, no dentist can tell you whether you have on going periodontal disease. A dentist can only tell you if you've had bone loss.

Not all changes in the bone that anchors the teeth are pathological changes. The trabecular bone is the spongy supporting bone that forms the core of the jawbones; the condition and density and trabecular pattern of bone all change as we get older. In addition, the ligaments get less flexible as we age. So if some bone loss and gum recession are caused by normal function and aging rather than by bacteria, we may be over treating periodontal disease. If periodontal disease is caused by an underlying medical condition, we may be over treating periodontal disease.

Removing teeth in elderly patients who have had sizable bone loss can be very difficult. The teeth may not come out easily. Why? Does the trabecular pattern of bone change to compensate for bone loss? Does the ligament, the PDL, become more hardened or calcified to compensate for bone loss? The human body compensates for changes that occur, or it adapts to changes in order to function better. If we lift weights, our bones become stronger. When we lose bone around our teeth, the bone and ligament holding the remaining teeth must get stronger. Ironically, periodontists never mention this type of compensation in any literature. They merely focus on bone levels. Why?

There are four types of bone in the human face, and the length of treatment for placing and restoring implants with a crown depends on which type of bone the implant is placed in. It is crucial that implants integrate with the surrounding bone before a tooth and crown are placed in that bone.

Type I bone is like the wood of an oak, which is very hard and dense. Therefore, it takes about five months for this type of bone to integrate with an implant.

Type II bone can be compared to pine wood, which isn't as hard as type I. It usually takes four months for this type of bone to integrate with an implant.

Type III bone is like balsa wood, which isn't as dense as type II. Normally it takes six months for this type of bone to integrate with an implant.

Type IV bone is comparable to Styrofoam, which is the least dense of all of the bone types. It takes about eight months for this type of bone to integrate with an implant.

The four types of bone help determine implant longevity and prognosis. Maybe these criteria should have been used in studies that treated periodontal disease and to determine the success of any treatment for periodontal disease as well.

Could bone loss in our jaws be similar to arthritis—inflammation, swelling, and destruction of joints? There is no single cause of arthritis. Overuse, autoimmune disease, infection, and symptoms of other diseases, such as gout, can cause arthritis. Osteoclasts, bone-resorbing cells, are involved both with arthritis destruction and with bone loss around our teeth. The diagnosis of bleeding gums may be like lupus; it is sometimes hard to distinguish active lupus from infection, just as it may be difficult to distinguish whether gums bleed due to dental plaque or something else going on in the body.

Unfortunately, the epidemiology of periodontal disease is lacking. It is lacking because we don't have adequate staging—that is, we lack a classification system for diseases that uses diagnostic findings to produce clusters of patients who need similar treatment and have similar expected outcomes. Every study uses different criteria to measure periodontal disease, which makes it hard to evaluate the merits of these studies' conclusions. No study deals with the attributes of bone, as a dentist must do when placing an implant. No study deals with guidance in individual patients. Very few studies look at the composition of dental plaque before and after treatment. Very few studies look at vitamin D levels in patients.

Periodontal literature says occlusion or malocclusion does not cause periodontal disease but may make it worse. How does occlusion make periodontal disease worse, but not cause it? The studies look at static and aesthetic components of occlusion—class I, class II, or class III. No studies deal with occlusal scheme—the type of guidance for periodontal patients. Why?

If we define periodontal disease as bone loss, then occlusion will cause periodontal disease because dynamic forces causes bone loss. *What's also important is how we define occlusion or malocclusion.* Angle's classification of occlusion is not important because Angle's classification is purely an aesthetic classification. Malocclusion should be classified by guidance and function.

The dental literature says that removable partial dentures can torque teeth. If not properly designed, the metal clasps that attach the removable partial dentures to the natural teeth will put forces on the teeth that will cause them to loosen up and come out. *There is no difference between a bad occlusion that may cause torquing and tipping of teeth or a poorly designed partial denture.* These affected teeth will come out because of bad occlusion or a bad partial denture. However, periodontists will say erroneously that periodontal disease caused the teeth to loosen up and come out.

Antirotation devices are placed in implants. Why? Because of occlusal forces. Occlusal forces can cause implant screws to loosen up. Occlusal forces cause many things to happen.

When should a tooth be extracted? When should a tooth be extracted because of bone loss? After 50% bone loss, 75% bone loss, or 90% bone loss? Actually, if a tooth is very tight and doesn't show any periapical pathology on x-ray—that is, any damage to the area around the tip of the root of the tooth—then why should that tooth be extracted? The tightness of a tooth should be the important factor in determining whether or not it should be extracted, not the amount of bone loss.

Inflammation. Calculus. Bleeding. Gingivitis. According to periodontists, periodontal disease is an infection that gets under the gum and causes inflammation, the process by which the body responds to injury or an infection. Inflammation then starts dissolving the jawbone that supports the teeth. Periodontists also believe that periodontal infection may also contribute to other medical conditions. So they tell patients that they have to remove the infection in the pockets around the teeth, and that sometimes requires surgery. The goal of removing this inflammation and the pockets of infection is an important one.

Why is inflammation bad? For periodontists, inflammation is bad because it leads to periodontal disease. However, I believe that inflammation is bad because it could raise C-reactive protein (CRP) and may cause bleeding gums, which can lead to dark teeth, anemia, and dark stools. If teeth are washed in blood, they are prone to staining. Inflammation may also raise blood pressure.

Laboratory evidence and findings from various studies suggest that inflammation is important in atherosclerosis, the process in which fatty deposits build up in the inner lining of arteries. CRP is one of the acute phase proteins that increase during systemic inflammation. It's perceived that testing CRP levels in the blood can assess the risk of cardiovascular disease.

Bleeding gums cannot be controlled if caused by an uncontrolled systemic problem or systemic disease. Natural processes such as puberty, menstruation, and menopause; hormonal problems; diseases such as diabetes; dietary problems; and habits such as cigarette smoking can cause inflammation. Periodontists believe that plaque causes inflammation around the teeth. But everyone has plaque, which is the bacteria-containing substance that collects on the surface of the teeth. However, does the quantity of plaque or the composition of plaque cause destruction? That is the important question.

Almost everyone produces calculus or tartar. Calculus is mineralized plaque. The most common place for calculus to form is on the lower anterior teeth, yet the lower anterior teeth are usually the last teeth to be lost.

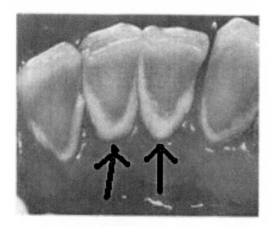

calculus

If this is the case, then we need to know whether plaque is distributed evenly over all the teeth or not. Do the lower anterior teeth have more plaque? We also need to know why the lower anterior teeth are the last to be lost even though they are more prone to calculus formation. And we need to know just how harmful calculus is.

While calculus is a nuisance, is it not that harmful if only a little bit remains? If calculus is so harmful, then the lower anterior teeth should be the first teeth to be lost, not the last. But the reality is that they are the last to be lost, and the reason is because they're not involved with either group function or balancing side function.

According to periodontists, gingivitis, which is caused by plaque buildup, is the mildest form of periodontal disease. But does gingivitis really have any relationship to periodontal disease? The answer is probably *no*. Although chronic gingivitis may exist in adults for long periods of times, no periodontal disease will necessarily develop. And although almost every adolescent who wears braces develops severe gingivitis, yet periodontal disease almost never occurs because of this inflammation. Why? Plaque retention is terrible when braces are worn, yet this plaque doesn't lead to periodontal disease!

We know that there are different types of inflammation found throughout the body. However, as dentists, we can't give a histological account of the inflammation that we see in gingivitis. Why?

There are also different types of plaque. The microbial composition of plaque varies between individuals and the location on the tooth. Periodontists believe that the composition of plaque, not the plaque itself, may be harmful. But if that's the case, why doesn't periodontal disease follow Koch's postulates? The reason is because something else is at play here—the host.

When the host is in a pathological or imbalanced condition, parts of the body break down. I believe the onset of severe periodontal disease at an early age is a precursor to an early death. Unhealthy people get periodontal disease. Unhealthy diet, lack of sleep, smoking, excessive drinking, and vitamin D deficiency all make one unhealthy. An undiagnosed medical condition, such as diabetes, will also cause periodontal disease.

In adolescence, children are usually healthy, and it is documented that older teenage boys have high levels of precursors of bone-forming cells circulating in their blood. This may be the reason why braces don't cause bone loss in youngsters.

6

Routine Treatment of Periodontal Disease

I'll be criticized by the dental profession for giving cookbook recipes to treat periodontal disease, just as I criticize periodontists for their cookbook treatments. As a starting point, in order to treat periodontal disease, the dental profession wants to eliminate pockets. What exactly is a pocket? A pocket occurs when the inner layer of the gum and bone pull away from a tooth and small spaces appear between the tooth and gums. These pockets collect debris and can become "infected."

There are two types of pockets. In gingivitis; the pocket is small and shallow; as the disease progresses, the pocket becomes larger and deeper. In periodontitis, the pocket is large and deep.

For several reasons, the dental profession wants to eliminate pockets: decreasing the amount of plaque under the gums, decreasing inflammation, and increasing the ease of cleaning the teeth.

That agenda might seem logical, but the problem is that the plaque hypothesis doesn't satisfy Koch's postulates. Experimentally, transferring plaque from one person to another through inoculation doesn't cause periodontal disease to develop in the inoculated individual. Is it because disease depends on the host, not the plaque?

How do you measure inflammation quantitatively? You can't. It is a subjective measure. There is no scientific way to measure inflammation. You can get inflammation even if you don't have any plaque. Severe inflammation without plaque is possible. Plaque doesn't have to be present for inflammation to occur. What's more, the most aggressive type of periodontal disease occurs with no inflammation. A patient can get a severe case of the disease with no inflammation.

But does inflammation mean that periodontal disease exists? The answer is a resounding *no*. If that is the case, is the elimination of inflammation a worthy goal? It is worthy, but not as important as we may be led to believe, in eliminating periodontal disease. Also, if it is not the amount of plaque but the composition of the plaque that matters, why do we worry about pockets?

Straight teeth are easier to clean, yet orthodontic studies show that crooked teeth are not lost any sooner than straight teeth. The connection between ease of cleaning and keeping one's teeth must be a fallacy.

How do we eliminate pockets? Do we have to subject patients to painful gum surgery just because that is the way periodontists have always eliminated pockets? No. Research indicates that over 20% of patients don't get any benefit from this treatment. In fact, they continue to lose teeth while undergoing this treatment. But even though there are nonsurgical procedures to eliminate pockets, the dental community is reluctant to upset the status quo, so gum surgery remains the treatment of choice.

Periodontists want to get rid of pockets by reducing inflammation, eliminating gum tissue, adding bone, and then removing teeth after surgery fails. Their next tactic is putting in dental implants.

The first phase of periodontal therapy, scaling and root planing, a method of treating pockets that are larger than three millimeters, should reduce inflammation, if not eliminate it. If pockets remain after scaling and root planing, dentists may want to remove gum or rearrange gum tissue to eliminate the pockets. They may also want to do regenerative procedures to bring back lost bone. Or they may want to extract the teeth and put in implants.

But there are consequences to eliminating or rearranging gum tissue. The gums will look receded. The teeth may become very sensitive to temperature. The teeth will be more prone to tooth decay and root caries. Food is more easily trapped in these spaces. The teeth may hurt for a very long period of time. The teeth will look longer. Some people call the effects of this procedure disfigurement; they don't like the look of receded gums.

In addition, periodontists might suggest bone or tissue grafts to replace or encourage new growth of bone or gum tissue. The bone grafts allow for the regeneration of new bone in an area where bone has been lost. But there are risks with this procedure. Since each case is different, it's not possible to predict accurately which grafts will be successful. Bone grafts may come from a patient's own bone, cadaver bone, bovine bone, or synthetic bone. A patient's own bone is optimal.

Periodontists might also remove a tooth to get rid of pockets and then place implants. But it might not be easy to add implants if there's not enough bone. In that case, bone grafts are again used.

Dental implant surgery, like any surgery, poses some health risks, including infection at the implant site; injury or damage to other teeth, blood vessels and the nasal cavity; nerve damage; and even sinus problems. For the most part, dental implant surgery is becoming very routine.

The most compelling reasons not to perform periodontal surgery came from data insurance companies refused to release. At the Yankee Dental meeting in Boston in 2007, a presenting dentist said that claims from insurance records showed that, contrary to popular wisdom, periodontal surgery does not save teeth. I asked this dentist if I could see the data, or if he could release the data, and he said that he could not. He explained away the claims of the insurance companies by saying that the periodontists were doing surgery on the most difficult cases or on the worse teeth, and that was why patients were still losing their teeth. Cases were failing because the dentists were choosing the wrong cases. This is an outrageous explanation or a coverup.

Occlusal equilibration

When our teeth and jaws do not occlude, or come together, in an acceptable position because they lack anterior or canine guidance or have protrusive interferences or have one tooth hit before all the others, dentists can usually correct the condition with occlusal equilibration. This condition can also be corrected with tooth movement (braces) or prosthetics (crowns).

Occlusal equilibration is the reshaping or recontouring of the surfaces of teeth. It can be done to make centric relation equal to centric occlusion. I don't think this is a good idea because of the possibility of developing sleep apnea. It can and should be used to eliminate prematurities, or instances where one tooth hits first before all the others. Many patients develop acute pain from prematurities. Occlusal equilibration can and should be used to eliminate group guidance and balancing side guidance.

A simple occlusal equilibration can be accomplished in a short time, while more complex equilibrations may require several appointments. It should be noted that most insurance companies do not pay for occlusal equilibration.

My cookbook treatment for periodontal disease

When I see a patient for the first time, I want to examine the areas of the mouth with bone loss. I then have to examine the area and determine if the bone loss came from occlusion, from being next to an extraction socket, from missing teeth, from orthodontic treatment, from eruption sequence, from decay, from the type of lifestyle the patient leads, from systemic disease or faulty dentistry or smoking.

If the patient has group or balancing side guidance or protrusive interferences, that condition must be removed, and the patient must be put into anterior or canine guidance.

The patient must then be fully scaled and root-planed. And then, if possible, the patient should be put on systemic antibiotics for three months and come back every three months for repeat treatment. Numerous studies by Sigurd P. Ramfjord, DDS, show scaling and root planing are as effective as any other treatment if done every three months. According to Ramfjord, surgery is seldom warranted, except in the rare cases of extremely advanced disease. Those cases can benefit from flap surgery in which the gum tissue is not removed, but placed aside for deep scaling and then stitched back into place.

Studies done with subjects with localized aggressive periodontitis (LAP) and generalized aggressive periodonitis (GAP), two very destructive periodontal diseases, show that systemic antibiotics can regenerate lost bone. This is why I prescribe antibiotics. Localized aggressive periodontitis (LAP) is characterized by severe and localized bone loss around the first molar and incisor teeth. Generalized aggressive periodontitis (GAP) usually affects people under thirty years old and affects at least three permanent teeth other than first molars and incisors. GAP and LAP are classifications of two types of most aggressive periodontal disease. GAP and LAP are rare.

Besides brushing, I advise the patient to use an oral irrigator, e.g., a water pick, at least once every day. Some studies show that using this device also restores lost bone. Patients may floss if they wish, but it is not a high priority. Flossing is only important if you eat certain foods, such as corn, roast beef, or chicken. Flossing may help to prevent tooth decay.

Antibiotics

Antibiotics have advanced medicine and dentistry over the last seventy years.

Antibiotics have saved an untold number of lives. Today, though, we take them for granted. But we don't take them for granted in dentistry. Many dentists avoid using them for periodontal therapy. These dentists argue that resistance to antibiotics can take place. Granted, resistance to antibiotics is a potential problem, but dentists and patients need to make choices and decide when to use them. If you can bring back bone by using antibiotics, why not use them?

Tetracyclines

Dermatologists have prescribed countless doses of tetracycline, an antibiotic used to treat a variety of bacterial infections. Tetracycline has been used for years to control acne. Some doctors advocate long-term use of tetracycline to cure Lyme disease. Some rheumatologists are giving long-term doses of the antibiotic to treat rheumatoid arthritis and other autoimmune diseases. Tetracycline is very safe when used as prescribed. And there have been no reported cases of any deaths from the use of tetracycline. I usually like my patients with bone loss to be on 250 milligrams of tetracycline, once a day, for a hundred doses. I may also prescribe doxycycline, another antibiotic in the tetracycline family. A patient who needs to be started on a three-month dental recall because of bone loss probably should start off with a three-month course of tetracycline.

Tetracycline, besides acting as an antibiotic, works in another most important way. It seems to prevent osteoclasts and osteoclast precursors from dissolving away bone. It prevents MMPs, osteolytic enzymes, from dissolving soft tissue and bone. Osteoclasts are the cells responsible for bone destruction anywhere in the body.

I also treat periodontal disease with other antibiotics, such as metronidazole and amoxicillin, but not on a long-term basis. Why? Because some studies show that these antibiotics can bring back lost bone when used for short periods of time.

Mouthwashes and anti-inflammatories

Mouthwashes and anti-inflammatories are an adjunct treatment, depending on hygiene, compliance, inflammation, and discomfort. I used to use Meclomen, a nonsteroidal anti-inflammatory drug. However, because it is a prescription drug, it is not as favored as the over-the-counter anti-inflammatory drugs.

7

Case Histories

The case study method is a great way for others to learn more about dentistry. I like to follow my patients so I can see how my treatment has worked out. Doing so has also influenced the way I see dentistry connected to the practice of general medicine.

As I follow my patients' progress, I sometime think that maybe I have a skewed practice because my patients seem to have different outcomes than what is expected. That is because, unlike the majority of the dental community, I have found that teeth are usually lost when a patient undergoes periodontal surgery. I don't know why data compiled from insurance claims records, demonstrating that periodontal surgery doesn't save teeth, isn't being released. I think maybe the dental community doesn't want the information released in order not to upset the status quo.

We often see ads touting the design of one toothbrush over another because if its ability to get rid of plaque. If we want to get rid of plaque, we pay attention to the toothbrush that is designed to accomplish that task. Now let's take that logic a step farther. If canine guidance is designed to make our mouths work best, why don't most dentists pay attention to guidance and occlusion?

It's because many dentists can't, or don't want to, see the trees for the forest. The primary reason is because dentists are not taught about occlusion in dental school. Dentists are more interested in doing a root canal than wondering why a tooth needs a root canal in the first place.

If you study landscape design, you study how the wind and soil will affect everything in the garden. You learn that strong trees will protect weak trees. You study water runoff and all the forces that affect the landscape. Well, a certain force affects the teeth. Occlusion is this force. We must study how the teeth are placed in our landscape, the mouth, in order to better treat and protect our patients.

Besides checking for cavities, a little investigation also allows dentists to diagnose any number of medical problems. For example, a dentist who sees thin teeth in a patient's mouth would probably determine that the patient suffered from acid reflux disease. That's because the acid causes teeth to erode. In addition, diabetes can cause case bleeding gums and bad breath. White spots in the gums could be a sign of oral cancer. Accelerated tooth loss could be a sign of osteoporosis, while red or inflamed gums could signal heart disease. And dentists know that erosion of the teeth could also be a sign of bulimia.

One of my most recent cases involves a patient whom I shall designate as E. W. I had not seen E. W. before, but her husband and sister-in-law told her to call me. When she finally did call me, she was frantic. She was in a lot of pain. Her mouth guard had broken. She needed it at night and during the day to relieve her bruxism and headaches. She had to be seen right away.

Bruxism is a serious dental condition in which a person grinds his or her teeth while sleeping. Bruxism can damage the teeth and jaws and cause a person to have headaches as well as a sore face. To prevent those problems, something has to be done to stop the tooth grinding.

Although there is no there is no guaranteed way to stop the grinding itself, a mouth guard prevents the person from damaging the teeth, even though it might not stop the actual grinding.

A dentist can custom-fit a mouth guard to treat bruxism, but people respond differently to mouth guards. Wearing a mouth guard helps some people stop grinding their teeth, but it makes other people grind their teeth even more. Sometimes a mouth guard can help a person at first, but then becomes less effective as time goes on.

After I talked to this patient, I knew she had to be seen right away. So I saw her and took her out of group guidance. Remember that in group guidance, all the pressure during lateral movements of the jaw is progressively borne by all the back teeth. And the teeth stop the lower jaw from hitting the upper jaw.

For the person with normal-sized jaws, the tips of the lower back teeth that are closest to the cheeks, the buccal cusps, should touch the centers of the upper back teeth when the jaw closes. These two areas should never be touched with the drill or ground down. This will prevent the vertical dimension of the face from getting smaller if the teeth need to be reshaped. Vertical dimension refers to the height of the face when the teeth are brought together. If the teeth are worn down or dentures are worn down, the vertical dimension of the face will be decreased. Decreasing the vertical dimension of your face will make you look older. Most often worn or old dentures cause a decrease in vertical dimension. People who have no teeth and who don't wear dentures will have a collapsed vertical dimension and will look much older.

To change guidance, some of the back teeth need to be reshaped. The back teeth are the teeth behind the canines—the molars and bicuspids. Usually the upper front cusps of the back teeth need to be lessened, if there is group guidance. If there is balancing side guidance, usually the upper inside cusps of the back teeth, the lingual or palatal cusps, need to be lessened.

So I carefully reshaped E. W.'s teeth to take her out of group guidance, so as not to decrease the vertical dimension of her face. As a result, her symptoms were relieved almost instantly. She has not worn the mouth guard since, and I have since done restorative work on her. It has been over one year since she had any problems.

T. D. is a patient I have been following for twenty years. She has been complaining of vague TMJ pain for many years. TMJ problems are related to the jaw joint. Because our muscles and joints work together, a problem with either one can lead to stiffness, headaches, ear pain, head pain, neck pain, clicking sounds and even locked jaws.

T. D. hated her teeth because of the pain. After examining her, I found she had anterior guidance; the teeth in between the canines, the incisor teeth rather than the canines, touched when her jaw moved from side-to-side. I gave her supportive therapy and told her to see her physician, who diagnosed her with fibromyalgia, a chronic illness that causes immense physical pain and debilitating fatigue and affects all the systems in the body.

I believe vague TMJ pain may be one of the early signs of fibromyalgia. We may be over treating TMJ disorders that are really fibromyagia related problems. Since both TMJ and fibromyalgia are so closely related, it's important that they are properly diagnosed. Today T. D. is being treated for fibromyalgia.

Another patient, R. F., came to my office about seven years ago. She, too, suffered from fibromyalgia. R. F. was unhappy with her previous dentist because of all the pain she had suffered as his patient. She underwent a root canal and then had a crown placed on that tooth.

All her teeth were very sensitive to cold and hot temperatures. I took her out of group function, and her pain was alleviated. Her mouth calmed down. About two years later, she felt comfortable enough about me to have me put in a fixed bridge to replace her missing upper second bicuspid. She had never wanted to have that work done because she worried about the pain that dental work might cause her. She had a fixed bridge performed on two virgin teeth—teeth that had no decay or fillings. She also needed root canals to reduce her sensitivity to hot and cold. She still has a problem with adjustment to ambient temperature, but that's one of the symptoms of fibromyalgia.

M. I. has been one of my patients for almost twenty years. About fifteen years ago, after I filled some small cavities, she complained of constant pain. M. I. had anterior guidance; the teeth in between her canines, her incisor teeth, rather than her canines, touched when her jaw moved from side-to-side.

She was getting prescriptions for eight hundred milligram doses of Motrin for three months from her physicians as well as from me. I told her that her pain response was not normal. I told her to see a neurologist. She did, and the neurologist ended up finding a pituitary gland tumor.

The pituitary gland is a small organ about the size of an acorn. The pituitary gland is located at the base of the skull and surrounded by a bony saddle-like structure above the sinuses at the back of the nose. The pituitary gland releases substances that control the basic functions of growth, metabolism, and reproduction.

Doctors also found that M. I. had high levels of prolactin because of this tumor. High levels of prolactin can cause low bone density.

At this time, her doctors have chosen to observe this tumor rather than operate. Whenever she visits me, she expects to have pain for weeks after dental treatment. I believe her pituitary tumor and the pain in her mouth are related.

D. R. was one of my early patients. I first started seeing her around 1981. I wanted to put white fillings on her upper front teeth, but her gums always bled. It is very hard to do white fillings if the gums bleed.

D. R. was a young woman whose gums bled profusely even though she didn't have any bone loss. I asked her to take tetracycline for two days before she came in for treatment. I had seen how systemic tetracycline stopped bleeding in many patients, so I thought it might work in her case. I put her on the tetracycline, and I did the fillings without a problem.

Later I learned that she was also on oral contraceptives. The oral contraceptives were probably responsible for her bleeding gums. Women who use oral contraceptives may be susceptible to the same oral health conditions that affect pregnant women, including red, bleeding, and swollen gums.

Today we know that antibiotics can lessen the effect of oral contraceptives, but we didn't know that when I first treated D. R. in the 1980s. I often wonder how the Federal Drug Administration put oral contraceptives on the market without knowing they could interfere with antibiotics! The important question is: Do antibiotics that interfere with oral contraceptives play the same role in preventing bone loss in periodontal disease by interfering with sexual hormones? Bone loss before puberty is almost nonexistent. Is the hormonal factor another clue to the way that tetracycline prevents bone loss?

T. N. is a dentist who practices outside of Boston. I have known him for over twenty years. About eight years ago, we were seated together to view a new type of dental equipment. He was a recent convert to Pankey Institute in Florida. He went down there and had his bite adjusted so his centric relation equaled his centric occlusion. I told him there was a danger in doing this because sleep apnea could develop. T. N. already had sleep apnea and used a CPAP machine. He denied that adjusting his bite caused him to get sleep apnea, even though it occurred after his bite was adjusted.

T. W. has been a patient of mine for about three years. She has no bone loss, and her occlusion is fine, but her gums always bleed profusely. She wanted her teeth to be cleaned every three months. Her former dentist agreed that frequent cleaning was probably a good idea because of all the bleeding. So he scheduled her for a cleaning every three months.

When I saw her, I put her on systemic tetracycline, but the drug didn't stop the bleeding. I then suggested that when she next saw her physician, she should ask him to test her for von Willebrand disease. Von Willebrand disease is an inherited bleeding disorder named after the doctor who discovered it, Erik von Willebrand. People born with the disease have low levels of a protein called von Willebrand factor that helps the blood to clot. When von Willebrand factor is missing or the levels are low, it can cause prolonged bleeding after an injury or accident. The symptoms of von Willebrand disease include unusual bruising, abnormal menstrual bleeding, bleeding in the mucous membranes, such as the gums and nose, and excessive or prolonged bleeding after a tooth is pulled.

T. W. didn't have von Willebrand's disease, but within a year she was diagnosed with breast cancer. She had surgery for the cancer, and she went through chemotherapy. I saw her recently, and her gums don't seem to bleed. Now I see her for cleanings every six months. I believe her cancer caused her gums to be inflamed and bleed. One wonders whether she had an imbalance in her body between estrogen and progesterone. Imbalances between these hormones can cause bleeding elsewhere in the body.

F. M. was one of my earliest patients, and I still see him today. He suffers from Type 1 diabetes. In Type 1 diabetes, which is a lifelong condition, the pancreas stops making insulin. Without insulin, the body is not able to use glucose or blood sugar for energy. For the rest of his life a person with Type 1 diabetes must inject insulin, follow a diet plan, exercise daily, and test his blood sugar several times a day.

F. M. was very strict and faithful about his diet and blood sugar all the time. About fifteen years ago, he came in for a routine cleaning, and his gums bled profusely. He had no bone loss. But because of the profuse bleeding, I put him on tetracycline, 250 milligrams, four times a day for two weeks, and asked him to return so I could clean his teeth again. When he came back two weeks later, his gums still bled profusely. I was really concerned. I didn't expect his gums to bleed.

We've known for quite a while that people with diabetes have an increased risk of developing severe periodontal disease. One study suggests that diabetics may have a problem with the maturation and function of osteoblasts, the cells responsible for bone formation throughout the body. Studies have shown that people with diabetes have more and deeper pockets between their teeth than other people. Type I diabetics have lower bone mass than normal people.

F. M.'s diabetes caused his gums to bleed even though his blood sugars were normal. In less than a month, he had a severe hemorrhage in one eye. His gums almost never bleed today, and he has a nice bone level around his teeth. I believe his bleeding gums then were the result of something going on throughout his whole body.

G. E. has been my patient for over twenty years. He has bone loss and missing teeth. His dental condition is pretty stable. I've been seeing him every three months for a number of years. One day last year while I was treating him, his gums began to bleed heavily. His gums seldom bleed. I asked him to take tetracycline. When I saw him three months later, his gums were great. They were tight, and there was no more bleeding. I asked him if he had taken the tetracycline I prescribed. He said no. However, he told me he had ended up in the hospital less than a week after I last saw him. He had diverticulitis and had been on intravenous antibiotics for a week. Those antibiotics did the trick. His bleeding gums were a symptom of his diverticulitis.

I first saw E. D. in 1981 when he was thirty-seven. He was not a smoker, but he was a little overweight. He was a regular patient who also had regular physical checkups as well. His gums were always very inflamed, but he had no bone loss. His gums would bleed profusely every time his teeth were cleaned, and he would often develop a high temperature after the cleaning.

Whenever people have their teeth cleaned or even when they brush regularly, bacteria enter the bloodstream. Until very recently, the American Heart Association felt that most people with heart murmurs should be premedicated with antibiotics before dental cleanings. Today the American Heart Association thinks that antibiotic premedication should be reserved mostly for patients who have had heart valve replacements. Many times I would place E. D. on antibiotics before a cleaning to prevent a rise in temperature after a cleaning. When he was fifty-nine, he developed a mild heart condition and needed bypass surgery. Just before his heart condition appeared, he developed a problem with his eyelids, a condition called blepharal spasm. Currently, botox treatments help keep his upper eyelids from closing. He still doesn't have any bone loss, but he still has swollen gums that continue to bleed when his teeth are cleaned. However, even though he often develops a temperature after his teeth are cleaned when not on antibiotics and even though his gums continue to bleed, he doesn't have periodontal disease. Also, no one knows the cause of blepharal spasm.

E. U. is a patient I saw last year for the first time. She is forty-four years old, suffers from a genetic blood disorder, smokes a pack of cigarettes a day, has a dry mouth from medicines she takes, is very heavy, and has scarring in her lungs from her clotting problem. She has severe bone loss around her upper teeth, and I have suggested a full plate.

Recently she came in to have a loose tooth removed. Later that week she saw her internist, and he did a vitamin D serum level test. Her vitamin D level was 9; a normal level is over 32. I then saw E. U. one month later to have another hopeless tooth extracted. After she had taken vitamin D for a month, her mouth had vastly improved. Her teeth had tightened up, and inflammation in her gums had almost disappeared. I had a hard time believing that this was the same patient I saw four weeks earlier. Are low vitamin D levels responsible for bone loss around the teeth? I think so. We know low vitamin D levels are associated with many other diseases, such as osteoporosis, and hypertension. Most doctors and many lay people acknowledge the body/mind connection; E.U.'s experience underscores the importance of the body/mouth connection.

A. S. was a patient of mine from 1988 until her death in 1995, at the age of eighty-six. She loved honey, and her son-in-law raised bees. I felt she had a higher rate of tooth decay because of her honey consumption.

A. S. had crowns on most of her teeth, but her lower right posterior bridge was broken. It had first been put in by another dentist in 1972 and was replaced in 1984 because it broke. I replaced it again in 1989. It broke again and had to be replaced in 1991. When it broke again in 1993, I replaced it at my own expense.

In 1993 her bridge split again. What was happening here? I discovered that this patient had a habit of biting extremely hard. The bridges did not chip, they split. On the second bridge I did in 1991, I went from using a gold alloy to using non-precious metal to make it harder and stronger. This is the only time I have ever used a non-precious metal in a crown and a bridge. And it broke again. Who would have thought an eighty-year-old woman had the jaw strength to break bridges? Forces are important in dentistry. Everything will break over time if the forces are hard enough.

B. N. was a patient of mine from 1990 through 1996. She left me in 1996 because I no longer accepted her insurance plan. In 1990 she was twenty-one years old and suffering from shortened roots on her upper front teeth. Her condition was probably caused by orthodontic treatment. I didn't have her previous x-rays, but she had the classic signs of shortened roots from orthodontic treatment. The roots of her two upper front teeth were about ¼ of an inch in length; they should have been about ¾ of an inch long. With such short roots, how did her teeth stay in place? Root shortening is a rare occurrence from orthodontic treatment. Forces applied from the braces sometimes cause the roots of the teeth to shorten. Teeth are held in the jawbone by their roots. If the root gets shorter, then there is less root to be held in by the jawbone, and thus the tooth is less able to withstand occlusal, chewing, or biting forces. Then, the tooth is more likely to be lost. My patient's condition showed the undesirable consequences of aggressive orthodontic treatment.

I first saw E. R. in 1988 because she suffered from chronic headaches and had vague pain in her face. She was thirty-five, and she suffered from Stickler syndrome, a genetic disease affecting the eyes, face, ears, heart, bones and joints. It is a connective tissue and collagen disorder. A person who suffers from Stickler syndrome typically presents with a distinctively flattened facial appearance, abnormalities of the eyes, hearing loss, and joint problems.

E. R. is also allergic to penicillin and mint. She had nice-looking crowns, but her bite was severely abnormal. She had severe balancing side guidance on both sides. Another dentist, a periodontist, had made her a mouth guard, which corrected her bite by eliminating the balancing side guidance. I ground down her back crowns so she would get anterior guidance and would not need her mouth guard anymore.

I still see E. R. She still gets headaches sometimes, but they're not as bad as they used to be. However, she doesn't have any acute pain in her TMJ joints. I don't know much about her illness, but I am surprised this collagen disease doesn't affect the teeth or the bone around the teeth. The good results of my treatment show that proper attention to guidance can relieve symptoms and improve function, even in patients with complex medical problems.

I first saw C. H. in 1994, when she was thirty-two years old and had cracked off her back upper right second molar. I sent her to an oral surgeon to have it removed. On that same day, I adjusted her bite and took her out of balancing side guidance. This guidance problem could have caused the tooth to crack. She also suffered from chronic, severe migraines. Adjusting her occlusion did not affect her migraines. In 2005 she was diagnosed with von Willebrand disease. Her gums have always bled when she had a cleaning, but she didn't suffer from any bone loss. As I mentioned before, von Willebrand disease is a blood disorder of varying severity. Up to 2% of the population may have this disease. I think her very severe migraines were related to this disease. She always had gingivitis but never had any bone loss. Dental work would also trigger her severe pain. She is now being treated for von Willebrand disease, has fewer migraines, and finds that dental work is much easier for her. From my practice, I feel dentists should be aware of the possibility of von Willebrand disease when a patient presents with severe migraines and bleeding gums.

S.C. has been a patient of mine for about five years. When I first saw him, I couldn't believe what I saw. His gums were extremely swollen and not well attached to the bone. I could touch his gums with a mirror and move them so easily that I could see the bone underneath the gums. Usually a dentist needs a scalpel or knife to cut the gums to see the underlying bone. The patient had bone loss, but not as much as you would expect with this condition. The patient bled profusely and, a physician was treating the patient. But what was he being treated for? The answer was too many bowel movements. Was swallowing so much blood causing the diarrhea? The patient also had balancing side and group function, which I corrected, and the patient was also put on antibiotics. Today, the patient's gums don't bleed, and he has normal bowel movements. He is also on a daily maintenance dose of tetracycline.

R. H. has been a patient of mine for about fifteen years. I have known his wife since we were teenagers. He comes in almost every six months for preventive care. About five years ago, his gums were inflamed. His gums bled profusely when his teeth were cleaned. He was developing bone loss on his posterior teeth. He had good occlusal guidance. I recommended he go on systemic tetracycline. After some pleading, he reluctantly agreed. One year later, he almost died. Doctors had to perform a triple bypass on his heart. He was not even fifty years old. Now his gums do not bleed. Since he has never smoked, I believe his bleeding gums and bone loss were the result of his heart condition. I believe that inflammation from his heart spread throughout his whole body. Abnormal conditions in the mouth can serve as advance warning of abnormal conditions elsewhere in the body.

A. V. has been a patient of mine for about ten years. She is about thirty years old, but she looks like a teenager. Her gums have receded throughout her mouth. She gets her teeth routinely cleaned. She was anorexic, and she went through a difficult time when she broke up with her daughter's father. When she was twenty-eight, I asked her to see her physician for a bone density scan. Her physician refused. She asked him a second time, and he relented. Because of her low bone density scan, she is now taking Fosamax. How many thirty-year-olds are on Fosamax? Very few. I believe her osteoporosis at an early age was responsible for her bone loss around her teeth.

A. L. has been a patient of mine for about eight years and is now about forty-six years old. When I first saw him, he had moderate bone loss. Scaling and root planing and systemic antibiotics were the treatments I prescribed. I also told him how important it was to use a water pick. He didn't come back to see me for three years; he finally came back because he had a toothache. He needed a lower back wisdom tooth extracted. He told me his water pick had broken two weeks earlier, and all of a sudden the tooth had started acting up. I made sure I took a full mouth set of x-rays on this patient so I could compare it with his older ones. His clinical exam looked excellent, and his new x-rays showed improvement. The bone grew back. I believe the water pick has kept his condition from deteriorating. He didn't come in for regular cleanings, so I have to assume that something was working to promote and stabilize his oral health.

D. T. was an early patient of mine who died last year. He was only fifty-four. He had suffered from Crohn's disease since he was a teenager. He also had poor nutrition because of a short intestine caused by intestinal surgery for Crohn's. Sometimes he developed ulcers in his mouth because of Crohn's disease.

He had periodontal surgery three times on the same teeth, plus multiple crowns and bridges that failed. He wore a denture for at least the last fifteen years of his life. I don't know what kind of occlusion he had. Early in my practice, I wasn't concerned about guidance, and I didn't find out. Guidance wasn't a topic taught in dental school back then, and no one talked about it when I was doing my dental internship either. If I had to treat D. T again, I would have made sure that he had canine or anterior guidance, and I would not have recommended periodontal surgery, especially not three times. I think his physical condition caused him to lose his teeth. Periodontal surgery accelerated their loss.

B. C. is a patient I treated for fifteen years until she remarried and moved away. Because she had colitis, she was often on prednisone.

Whenever her colitis was out of control, her gums were out of control. Scaling and root planing would never bring her inflammation around her teeth under control when her colitis was out of control. She could not take antibiotics because they would wreck havoc with her bowels. She continued to lose bone, and I told her she would probably lose her teeth unless her colitis was controlled.

D. H. is a current patient of mine, at least when she decides to come in. But she only comes in the morning because she isn't sober in the afternoon. Her physician tells me she drinks constantly. Her husband told me when I first started treating her that she was an alcoholic. She would go through a quart of hard liquor in a weekend. She comes in sporadically. I've asked her to see other dentists to get a biopsy of her gum tissue, but she hasn't done that. I think she has scurvy, which is a deficiency of vitamin C. Symptoms of scurvy include nausea, weakness, loss of hair and teeth. Scurvy can be fatal. Today, scurvy is a very rare disease, most often found in alcoholics. A few years back, my patient did end up at a periodontist's office, although I didn't know she was going. I wish the periodontist had done a biopsy then. Later that day, the periodontist called me and wanted to know what was up with the patient. "Alcohol," I told him, and he understood.

D. H. bruises easily and is very thin. I have had the opportunity to observe her gum condition for many years. Scaling and root planing have no effect on her tissues. Once I had her on vitamin K therapy, but I really don't like to prescribe vitamin K. It's very hard to treat an alcoholic medically. Her inflammation and severe gingivitis is due to a vitamin deficiency. Any gum treatment any dentist could offer her will be doomed to failure because of her underlying medical condition.

J. E. is a patient I have seen for over twenty-five years. He is about sixty years old. I think I first saw him on New Years Day of 1982. He had a history of acute periodontal abscesses on different teeth. He had no pocketing and little bone loss. His teeth were very firm, although he was missing some teeth. His gums were very tight. He never had inflammation of the gums, but he would often get these periodontal abscesses. Multiple periodontal abscesses, without pocketing, are rare. Was he doing something to cause this problem, or did some physical condition cause his abscesses? After a systemic course of tetracycline, however, he never had abscesses again. Although J.E.'s case was complex, his excellent response to systemic tetracycline followed the pattern I have observed in many of my patients.

J. E. had a history of testicular cancer. He also complained constantly about pain in his mouth and upper face. About ten years ago, I replaced an upper missing tooth with a bridge. A few years later, the bridge failed because his canine tooth cracked. It's very rare for a canine to crack, and his was one of the thickest and longest canines I have seen. Recently the patient asked to have a full upper set of dentures. He didn't want implants or a partial denture, but full upper dentures. His wife has had full dentures for forty years, and now it was his time. He figured that maybe if he had the teeth out, the pain in his upper face would go away. So we planned to do upper dentures immediately. I removed the teeth.

I've extracted my fair share of teeth, and his teeth did not come out easily. A lot of bone came out with the teeth—something that almost never happens. Were there hairline cracks in the bone that caused him to have pain all the time? I knew he had a very hard bite. We know hairline fractures in wrists, hips and ankles can cause pain, so I think there was a possibility that he had a hairline fracture in his upper jaw. He closed his mouth so hard that his canine cracked, so why not the bone in his face?

My patient has another idiosyncrasy. Novocain, the common dental anesthetic, has very little effect on him. He also can't wear jewelry, especially non-gold jewelry, because it makes his skin turn black. It seems that Novocain doesn't work well with patients who have skin allergies to metals. I used Marcaine, a long-acting local anesthetic, when treating him. From J. E., I have learned to ask patients who don't respond typically to Novocain if they have problems wearing metal jewelry.

D. D. and G. H. are two interesting patients who are now both deceased. D. D. came into my office in 1986 with severe bone loss. She was overweight, forty-one years old, and a smoker. She had no history of high blood pressure or diabetes. She did have tuberculosis as child and had been hospitalized for it. She had many areas of deep pocketing and many loose teeth. After I had been seeing her for four months, I extracted her upper teeth and inserted an upper plate. Four years later, I extracted many of her lower teeth and immediately inserted a lower partial plate. In 1991, at the age of forty-six, she died suddenly at home of a ruptured abdominal aortic aneurysm.

G. H. came into my office in 1996. He was forty-nine years old, of normal weight, and a smoker. His upper teeth were very loose. He had very severe bone loss with deep pocketing. His teeth were scaled and root-planed, and he was advised to have an upper denture placed. He refused because he didn't want to lose any more teeth. In eighteen months, he had to have an emergency denture placed because his upper bridge came out with his teeth attached. In December 2001, at the age of fifty-four, he suffered an abdominal aortic aneurysm and died three days later.

Death at forty-six and fifty-four years old respectively from an abdominal aortic aneurysm is very rare. Usually abdominal aortic aneurisms usually occur in old age. I feel that it is more than a coincidence that my two patients, D. D. and G. H., who died from abdominal aortic aneurysm, also suffered from severe bone loss around their teeth. The extent of these two patients' bone loss was striking and memorable. I may see no more than one or two patients a year who have so much bone loss around their teeth. I believe that severe bone loss may be a red flag that should prompt medical screening for systemic diseases to facilitate early detection and treatment.

J. D., age forty-one, also suffered from severe bone loss. He came into my office in 1986. He was married to D. D., mentioned above. Back then I wondered if he had caught some bad bacteria from his wife because he, too, had so much bone loss. I also wondered if periodontal disease was a communicable disease. If bad bacteria cause the condition we call periodontal disease, shouldn't husbands and wives or other people who have mouth-to-mouth contact infect each other? Wouldn't we see more "periodontal disease" in spouses? No studies have shown such a result. The bacteria in plaque that casues tooth decay is transmissible, but periodontal plaque is not. J. D. died in 2002, at the age of fifty-six, from brain cancer. Does a weakened immune system cause bone loss and cancer?

S. F. came into my office in 1990, at the age of thirty, suffering from severe bone loss. He died of a rare cancer within six years, leaving a small child. Did a weakened immune system cause both his cancer and bone loss? What is the periodontal condition of patients who die of cancer at an early age?

R. R. was an early patient of mine. I started seeing him in the early 1980s. He suffered from severe bone loss. He would cower when he had his teeth scaled. He died at forty-three of cardiac arrest. I now believe that his heart condition was related to his periodontal condition. He was a smoker. I would like to see a study of sudden deaths of people in their forties and their periodontal condition.

N.T. came into my office around 1986. She suffered from severe periodontal disease. Her breath was foul. Her teeth were all loose. I removed all her teeth and discovered she had almost no bone around any of her teeth. A short time later, she was diagnosed with diabetes, and within three years she died from cardiac arrest. She was about forty-eight. Did her diabetes contribute to both her periodontal condition and her heart condition? I think so.

F. M. was also a patient of mine for two years. He suffered from severe periodontal disease. A smoker, he died of lung cancer at fifty-two. Did his immune system fail him? I think so.

J. W. came into my office in 1993, when he was forty-two. He had severe bone loss. His teeth were scaled and root-planed. He didn't want any teeth removed. He had a lower Maryland bridge placed on his lower front teeth.

A Maryland bridge is used when there are healthy teeth on both sides of the space left by a missing tooth. However, unlike conventional fixed bridges, the Maryland bridge does not require the use of crowns or extensive tooth preparation. The bridge is bonded to the teeth abutting the space.

This was the only time a consultant from the patient's insurance company called me to question my procedure because the patient had so much bone loss. I told the consultant that the patient wanted a lower Maryland bridge. The insurance company paid for the procedure. This patient died three years later of a sudden heart attack. J. W. was yet another patient who died early of heart disease and who had severe periodontal bone loss.

J. M. came into my office in 1981 when she was thirty-three. She had had her gums cut by her previous dentist. She showed moderate to severe bone loss. Ever since her gum surgery, she had suffered severe pain when her teeth were cleaned. Many times she would have to go on narcotics after having her teeth scaled and root-planed. She was also a smoker, and she died of lung cancer around 2002. Why did she die at such an early age? What is the periodontal condition—bone loss—of patients who die at an early age?

T. G. is a diabetic and is forty-four years old. I have been treating him for thirteen years. He lost an upper front tooth many years ago, and he wore a flipper, a one-tooth removable denture, for many years. A flipper is also sometimes called a stay plate.

I wanted to do a traditional bridge, but the patient couldn't afford it. We then decided to do a Maryland bridge because that option costs less. A Maryland bridge is a false tooth that is cemented to adjacent teeth with a metal backing. But just as we decided to do that procedure, his gums got really inflamed, and pus came out of his pockets on two of his upper front teeth. Also, the teeth were loose.

So I cut his gums and placed him on systemic tetracycline. I also felt that if he was on tetracycline long enough and his diabetes was under control—he told me it wasn't under control—the issues with his gums would resolve. Also, maybe the splinting of his loose teeth by the Maryland bridge would improve his condition.

Over the course of the last ten years, I have had to re-cement the bridge three times. Today, T. G. is waiting for a kidney transplant. He vomits daily. Because of all the acid damage from the daily vomiting, the teeth that hold the Maryland bridge have shrunk in size, but the bridge is still firm. Who would have thought the bridge would remain tight and that his bone level wouldn't change? His diabetes is under control, but his life is tenuous. I am surprised that he hasn't lost any more bone.

N. D. is a forty-seven-year-old woman. I have been treating her for the last seven years. When N. D. first came in, I learned that she ground her teeth, so I removed her from group guidance and put her into anterior guidance. After that she stopped grinding her teeth totally.

About a year ago, she called me just after she returned from a vacation, complaining of pain in her mouth. At that point I hadn't seen her in nine months, and she just called me out of the blue and wanted immediately to be seen. She told me some doctor thought she was mentally ill and wanted her to see a psychiatrist. She thought she had contracted parasites while she was on vacation. She wanted my opinion.

When she came in, I noticed how thin she was. It seemed she had lost about fifty pounds. She looked like she wore a size two rather than the size eight she had probably taken the last time I saw her. She wanted to show me her eye, which was completely red. She also showed me her hands and her feet. That day she was wearing sandals, which was unusual. In the thirteen years I had known her, I had never seen her wear anything except high heels.

When I looked at her, I noticed that the tips of her fingers and toes were bulbous. She also told me she had sores in her vagina. She asked me to look at her gums because they were sore. Her teeth were dirty from years of smoking. She had two large canker-like sores on her gums, encompassing the first and second molars of her upper teeth. The lesions were a light yellow. They were well defined.

An aphthous ulcer or canker sore is a type of ulcer, a painful open sore inside the mouth. It's caused by a break in the mucous membrane. Canker sores are never found on the gums or hard palate. They are usually found on mucosa, the thin tissue that lines the inside of the mouth.

Well, I told the patient that I thought she might have Behcet's disease, an autoimmune disease. Behcet's disease generally begins when people are in their twenties or thirties, but it can happen at any age. Symptoms of Behcet's disease include recurrent ulcers that look like canker sores in the mouth as well as on the genitals, and eye inflammation.

The disease can also cause various types of skin lesions, arthritis, bowel inflammation, and meningitis. Behcet's is a multisystem disease that can involve all the organs and affect the central nervous system, leading to memory loss and impaired speech, balance, and movement.

When I told N. D. about this possibility, she was relieved because at least she knew she wasn't going crazy. I told her to see a rheumatologist. Two weeks later, when I got back from vacation, the rheumatologist called me. He told me Behcet's was a rare disease and that he saw maybe one or two cases in a decade.

Remember, Behcet's disease generally affects the mouth, skin, and genitals. Why these three areas? Why do afflicted patients get inflammation of the blood vessels in these areas? Behcet's disease is an autoimmune disease, with no known blood test. And why does it always affect the mouth? We don't know.

R. G. is eighty years old. I have been treating him for twenty-four years. About thirty years ago, he lost a finger to an infection he developed after a fishing hook nicked his finger. When I first saw him in 1983, he had a nine-millimeter pocket between his upper right back molars. All dentists are taught that nine-millimeter pockets are bad. I put him on systemic tetracycline when I first saw him with that pocket.

For the first ten years that I treated him, he was on and off systemic tetracycline. After he retired, he moved to Florida for the winter months. I told him to see a dentist while he was in Florida to have his teeth cleaned. I wanted him to have his teeth cleaned often, at least every three months if possible. While he was in Florida, he saw three dentists; each one told him he either needed to have a tooth extracted or he needed periodontal surgery. He called me from Florida, and I told him not to submit to either procedure because neither one was necessary. The patient listened to me and put his trust in me. He had known me since I was a child. For the last five years, I have put him on systemic tetracycline regularly, one 250-milligram pill a day. He has seen numerous physicians in the last five years, and they have all said it's acceptable for him to be on tetracycline. All his teeth are as firm as they were in 1983, and his bone level has stayed the same. And now there is only a seven-millimeter pocket between the molars. His x-rays show no change over this period. This patient is prone to infections. How many people, after all, have lost a finger to an infection? Now he uses an electric toothbrush and a water pick in addition to taking the systemic tetracycline.

I feel that he would have lost his teeth if he had had periodontal surgery. Today, if he were to see a new dentist, I believe that dentist would probably recommend removing the tooth and replacing it with an implant. But would such a step be necessary?

P.T. has been a patient since 1985. Now she is fifty-five years old. She is a clencher with a capital C. She knows she clenches her teeth. She clenches to relieve her stress. But she doesn't grind her teeth while awake and doesn't grind her teeth while she sleeps. She wore a mouth guard at one time but won't wear one today. She has broken two bicuspids because of this clenching. Bicuspids are the most likely to be lost if they are broken. Both bicuspids had crowns—crowns help prevent teeth from cracking and splitting. Forces from clenching have ruined her teeth. She does not get headaches, only broken teeth.

B. W. came to my office four years ago when he was fifty-one. He had moderate to severe bone loss, and there was tons of tartar over all his teeth. He used to be a smoker, but he had quit ten years earlier. He had full mouth debridement and scaling and root planing, and he was placed on systemic tetracycline and Flagyl, another antibiotic.

I told him to come back to see me every three months, but he never did because he lost his dental insurance. He would have been a candidate for periodontal surgery by the standards of almost every periodontist. Well, he finally came back to see me four years later because he had insurance again. He told me he thought he chipped a filling in the back of one of his upper teeth. Well, I examined him but didn't see any chipped filling. However, I noticed that a piece of tartar had fallen off. Again, he had so much tartar that it was hard to see his teeth. His teeth were cleaned, and x-rays showed that there was no change in the bone levels of his teeth or pocketing in his gums. Over four years his condition has stabilized without any periodontal treatment, let alone surgery. Did he need surgery then? No. Does he need it now? I don't think so.

C. W. came into my office two years ago. She was fifty-three and married to B. W. She had no remaining upper teeth and only three remaining lower teeth. The three teeth were hopeless because there was so little bone. Two teeth were extracted, and one was left to help hold her lower removable partial. We would wait on the last tooth. She returned two years later because she had gotten dental insurance, and I had to extract that last tooth. I was surprised it lasted two years.

C. W. and B. W. have a lot of bone loss. Is their bone loss related? Do they harbor the same bacteria or have the same diet or have the same lifestyles? What is the epidemiology of couples having severe bone loss? Is it a coincidence? Is it because of smoking? C. W. and B. W. quit smoking about ten years ago. Will implants work in C.W.? I think they will work.

D. K. is another person who suffers from fibromyalgia. Temperature always affects her teeth. I expect all patients with fibromyalgia to need more time in the dental chair with pain management.

I first saw A. T. in 1987, when she was seventy. Today she's almost ninety. I hadn't seen her for the past two years. But recently she came in to see me. She told me she had had a fall and was on a lot of new medications. And now she had extensive cavities between her teeth. She has a dry mouth. A dry mouth can wreck havoc, causing rampant decay.

Controlling tooth decay is now a major problem for A. B. Her gums bleed, but she doesn't have any new bone loss, just decay. I prescribed heavy doses of fluoride for A. B. The patient is also on coumadin, a blood thinner, so I expect her gums to bleed when I clean them. Blood thinners cause the gums to bleed.

P. W. is thirty-three years old. She has been suffering from headaches for most of her life. She has a Type III occlusion with open bite and group and balancing side guidance. Remember, a Class III occlusion occurs when the lower jaw is bigger than the upper jaw. When I was on vacation, she saw another dentist who was covering for me, and he recommended a mouth guard for her. She bought one at the drug store, and she said it helps with her headaches.

I suggested she might want to have surgery to correct her jaws, but she said she no. She also told me she lost her orthodontic retainer last year, after which a space developed between her upper front teeth. I wish I had seen her before she had orthodontic treatment so that I could compare her status before and after treatment. I also wonder if her lost orthodontic retainer had acted as a mouth guard. I believe her open bite with group and balancing side guidance causes or contributes to her headaches.

D. M. is a patient I saw for another dentist a few months ago. She has the same bite as P. W. D. M. came in because a crown needed to be cemented. I asked her if she had headaches, and she said, "How do you know? I have been to countless doctors. No one knows why I get them."

D. M. is thirty-seven years old. I told her to return to her dentist and try a mouth guard to see if it might help with her headaches. I also told her that orthognathic surgery might work. These types of bites, such as P. W and D. M. have, are rare. Class III open bites are rare. I don't know why someone doesn't do a comprehensive study on these patients and examine their headaches.

C. I. is a patient I recently saw for the first time. She is sixty-eight years old. She has normal-sized jaws with group and balancing side function. I asked her to move her jaws from right to left and left to right, but she couldn't do it. I find this inability is very typical for many patients who have had group and balancing side guidance for many years. I had to force her jaws to do this movement, and that's when I discovered her group and balancing side guidance. I immediately changed her guidance into anterior guidance. After only about five minutes of re-shaping her upper back teeth, she immediately gained more movement of her jaws. This is the typical scenario. But what is also unusual about this patient is that she suffers from a great deal of bone loss in only two places: the palate region of her upper first molars. The gingival recession on these palatal molars is quite severe. Why there and nowhere else? Is it due to her occlusion? It can't be from brushing too hard.

At age ten, D. D. had his front tooth knocked out while playing street hockey. It was replanted—put back into the extraction socket—three hours later. A silver point root canal was performed out-side the mouth before replantation. For the next thirty years, at differ-ent times, a draining fistula occurred in the gum above the reimplanted tooth. The fistula was caused by the patient's body rejecting the tooth. At twenty-five, the patient was seen at a dental school in Boston by pro-fessors of endontontics, or root canal specialists, and all of them recom-mended extraction. The professors claimed there was no choice. The tooth must go. At age forty-nine, D. D. had a procedure done to remove half the root. After the root amputation, the fistula went away, and D. D. underwent Invasialign treatment—orthodontic movement without braces. Today the tooth is firm, with no fistula. The roots of adult or permanent teeth that have been avulsed, or knocked out of one's mouth, and then replanted, have a tendency to resorb. It is believed that when the PDL (periodontal ligament) is damaged, the body no longer recognizes the tooth as one's own tooth, but reacts to the tooth as to a foreign object. The body then tries to reject the tooth by destroying both the root and bone around the root. The root resorbs, and bone is damaged around the root that is being eaten away.

Dental implants work by fooling the body. Somehow the body doesn't recognize the titanium dental implant as a foreign body, but the body will reject a natural tooth that has a damaged PDL or no PDL. Is periodontal bone loss around an intact tooth caused by damage to the PDL? Is the same mechanism that causes a root to resorb at play? Does calculus slowly injure the PDL by mechanical encroachment? Can bacteria injury the PDL? Do mechanical forces injure the PDL? I think the answer to all of the above is "Yes."

8

What I Want from an Orthodontist

When I refer a patient to see an orthodontist, what finished results do I want?

Canine guidance if possible; if not, then anterior guidance, but with no protrusive interferences and no group guidance (group function), and no balancing side guidance!

- No open bite
- Full lip profile—no concave upper lip
- A pretty smile
- No edge-to-edge occlusion
- No spaces between the posterior teeth
- If possible, no spaces between the anterior teeth
- No rotations of teeth, no deep bite
- No protrusion, no root reabsorption of the teeth—this condition can only be seen with x-rays
- No extractions if possible
- No crowding of teeth
- Proper midline of teeth

- No more than two years of treatment
- No unilateral cross-bite, a condition that occurs when the top teeth bite inside the lower teeth and can occur with the front teeth or back teeth
- No extractions of any canine teeth
- Straight teeth with an adequate over-jet, the horizontal projection of the upper teeth beyond the lower
- No receding gums
- No cavities or spotting on the teeth around the braces
- Nice angulation of teeth, with adequate over-jet

How about Class III bites? Is a Class III bite acceptable? Yes, as long as there is no group or balancing guidance (function), and the patient is happy with how the patient looks. Appearances are subjective, not objective.

9

Contradictions in Dentistry

There are some contradictions in dentistry that I think everyone should be aware of.

- When lower gums recede, the treatment of choice for many periodontists is to add gum tissue to this area. So where there were no pockets, now there are pockets. Even though periodontists say pockets are bad, they appear to find it acceptable to make pockets so the patient will look better.

- The dentists who claim that amalgam fillings are unsafe because of the mercury they contain do not inform patients that white fillings may contain benzene and formaldehyde, that sealants may contain estrogen-like substances, and that white crowns may contain aluminum.

- Most dentists themselves have gold crowns, yet they push white crowns on their patients. That's because it's easier to persuade people to have white crowns than gold ones.

- If implantologists say occlusion is so important for implants, why isn't occlusion just as important for natural teeth? I say it is.

- Some dentists don't advocate the probing of implants; they just take x-rays to monitor implants. However, it would be considered negligence not to probe a patient's natural teeth.

- Deep pockets, which dentists claim contain more plaque, are not more prone to tooth decay, but shrinking pockets, which contains less plaque, make the teeth more prone to decay.

10

Questions to Ponder

An avulsed tooth, one has been knocked out, can often be reimplanted. And there's a good chance if it was stored properly in milk, saline, or saliva and reimplanted within an hour, the supporting tissues will reattach and hold the tooth in place, even though the nerves and blood vessels can't be repaired. Putting the tooth back in place is a pretty simple procedure. The dentist will clean the debris from the tooth socket with water and then slip the tooth back into place. He or she may splint it to the adjacent teeth with plastic resin and orthodontic wire to keep it stable so it can heal and reattach. However, a reimplanted tooth does not always reattach. If it doesn't reattach properly, the tooth may fuse to the jawbone or be reabsorbed into the body. This process occurs slowly. The dentist will monitor this condition and may also suggest further treatment such as a root canal.

Often, though, the body will reject the root or part of the root after re-implantation. Why does a root suddenly become a foreign body? It seems that the PDL prevents the body from responding to the root as if the root is a foreign object. When a root becomes a foreign object, the root and the bone around the root get reabsorbed. This reabsorption is usually a very slow process. Is periodontal disease really a disease in which the PDL gets damaged, and this damage causes just reabsorption of bone, not of a tooth? It seems that damage to PDL by occlusal forces, by bacterial insult, or by mechanical means such as tartar, over brushing, or overhangs (long fillings) is responsible for bone loss.

Another phenomenon we don't understand is why, when natural teeth are connected to dental implants, the natural tooth usually intrudes into the bone over a period of time. This is the reason that we don't connect natural teeth to implants.

Other questions to ponder include these.

- Why does periodontal disease begin at puberty? Do sex hormones play a role in bone loss? Is this how antibiotics work—by interfering with sex hormones?

- Why do the roots of baby teeth resorb when an adult tooth erupts, with no harm to the adjacent teeth?

- Why do most patients with severe periodontal disease not get severe tooth decay and why do most patients with severe decay not get severe periodontal disease?

11

Misconceptions in Dentistry

The following are some misconceptions in dentistry that we need to do away with.

Plaque causes periodontal disease. No. The body destroys itself with its immune system, or an imbalance occurs between the bone-forming cells and the bone-destroying cells.

Plaque follows Koch's postulates with periodontal disease. No. Plaque does not follow Koch's postulates because bacteria aren't present in every case of the disease, bacteria can't be isolated from the host with the disease and grown in a pure culture, plaque can't be reproduced when a pure culture of the bacteria is inoculated into a healthy susceptible host, and the bacteria isn't recoverable from the experimentally infected host.

Aggressive forms of periodontal disease have lots of plaque and calculus. No. Aggressive forms have little tartar and little plaque.

Because plaque causes tooth decay, we think it causes periodontal disease. No. It doesn't. Bacterial acid causes tooth decay.

Plaque is usually harmful. No. It probably protects the teeth. Plaque keeps fungus away. Are infants without any teeth more prone to fungal infections because they don't have a reservoir of plaque around their teeth? Why are denture wearers more prone to fungal infections? Because they don't have teeth? Why do fungal infections, rather than rampant periodontal destruction, occur in many types of immunosuppressed patients? AIDS patients are more likely to get fungal infections than bone loss. Dental plaque probably keeps fungal infections in check.

Most teeth are lost due to periodontal disease. No. Where is the epidemiology to prove this? The decision to remove teeth is subjective. In the 1980s, hospital dentists were telling insurance companies that teeth needed to be extracted because of "periodontal disease." But the real reason was that their patients wanted dentures.

Occlusion doesn't cause disease or periodontal disease. Well, if you define periodontal disease as the result of bone loss because of bacteria, then no. Tipping forces are destructive. Ask any orthodontist. Twisting forces are destructive. Ask any orthopedist. Overuse any part of the body, and damage occurs. The teeth are no exception. Occlusion can cause disease. Wear and tear causes tissue destruction, whether it is hard tissue or soft tissue.

Dentists have all the answers. No, we really don't.

All bacterial organisms are harmful. When they are at the wrong place at the wrong time, or all the time, perhaps so. However, *E. coli* bacteria are found in the digestive tracts of most humans and many animals. Usually these colonizations are beneficial, but they're harmful in other areas of the body. Syphilis and salmonella are always harmful. We forget this distinction. The organisms in plaque may not be harmful if they don't cause any disease.

Dental implants are better than natural teeth. No. There is no panacea in life or in the mouth. Implants have no ligament surrounding them, as teeth have. The periodontal ligament acts as a shock absorber, but implants have no shock absorber. Teeth are dynamic; they move. Implants are static; they don't move. Teeth decay; implants do not. Bone loss will occur around implants and around teeth. Bone loss around implants goes circumferentially, around teeth, in dribs and drabs.

Occlusion is important for implants and for teeth. Is occlusion more important for implants because an implant doesn't have a periodontal ligament as its shock absorber? Implants will fail, or loosen up, all at once; teeth will not. Implants cannot move; teeth can and will move. Gums can be inflamed around both implants and teeth. It takes months for an implant to be incorporated into bone. Implants should not be placed where the jaw is still growing. Bone has to be healthy for implants to work. Diseases of the bone will affect implants. Gingival tissue around implants will not grow as high as it will around teeth because of blood supply. The periodontal ligament around teeth contains a blood supply that helps the gingival tissue grow. Therefore it is better to place an implant next to a tooth than to have two implants next to each other.

Teeth will flex more than implants. The jawbone flexes less as we get older. The strength of bone-to-implant interface cannot be clinically assessed. We can move teeth and assess that movement on a scale of zero to three. Radiographic examination and mobility tests are the most reliable parameters in assessing dental implants, not dental probing. The dental profession thinks dental probing around teeth is more important than radiographic exams and that it is malpractice if this dental probing is not done.

Some dentists claim that implants are better than bridges because bridges are like large overhangs around teeth. Yet platform shifting used on implants for better gingival appearance is an overhang on an implant. Platform switching means using an abutment that is larger than the implant.

12

Some Studies I Would Like to See Done

- The life expectancy of patients who suffer severe bone loss around their teeth, not caused by occlusion, at ages thirty, forty, fifty, and sixty. How much bone loss, at least 40% in 40% of their teeth, or at least six millimeters of bone loss on 40 % of their teeth, do they have at these ages? If someone has very long teeth, is bone loss as important? If so, is it important with respect to keeping the teeth or as an indicator for health? The body does compensate for bone loss around teeth. In my practice, there are few patients who suffer this much bone loss, and the ones who have, generally, do not live to the age of fifty-five. Thank goodness, I don't see many of these patients. But I'd like to know why that's the case.

- Do patients with multiple sclerosis, an unpredictable disease of the central nervous system, thought to be an autoimmune disease, and patients with abdominal aortic aneurysms have more bone loss that's not caused by occlusion than other people? My patients with those diseases seem to have more bone loss.

- Do patients who were treated with long-term tetracycline for skin problems have less bone loss? Does tetracycline offer long-term protection against bone loss?

- What kind of occlusion and guidance do dentists find in patients who are eighty years of age or older and have all their teeth?

- What is the periodontal condition of newly diagnosed patients with very low vitamin D levels?

- How much gum recession do patients who have a severe Class III bite have? These patients have no guidance; they can't move their jaws from left to right. They should have less gum recession and less periodontal disease on most of their teeth.

- I would like to select a group of patients who present with canine guidance, anterior guidance, and group guidance. I would like to have them followed every year for ten years. I'd like to document what happens to their teeth during that period.

13

Tooth Decay in a Nutshell

Good epidemiology exists for tooth decay and the plaque that causes tooth decay. For decay, you need cariogenic plaque, a substrate (carbohydrate), and a tooth. Pretty simple. Since we can't eat and brush our teeth at the same time, some fermentation of food by plaque has to occur. Some acid has to be produced. This acid will attack the tooth and destroy minute parts of the tooth. Over time, these minute parts add up, and teeth will be destroyed. Saliva, however, comes to the rescue. Saliva helps repair or remineralize these minute parts of the tooth destroyed by acid.

Decay depends on plaque, food, the tooth itself, and remineralization. If you have plaque in your mouth that doesn't produce acids, you can't get tooth decay. The composition of the plaque and the quantity of plaque determine if you get tooth decay. Cariogenic plaque is the term for plaque that causes tooth decay. *Streptococcus mutans* and *lactobacillus* are the two primary bacteria found in plaque that causes tooth decay. They follow Koch's postulates. If you have high levels of cariogenic plaque, watch out.

I feel that patients who eat a lot of yogurt or take acidophilus, because they both contain high levels of *lactobacillus*, may be prone to higher levels of tooth decay. If you don't eat cariogenic food, there is a low chance that you will get tooth decay. Cariogenic foods are carbohydrates that are fermented by cariogenic bacteria. If you are on the low-carbohydrate Atkins Diet, you are probably less likely to have tooth decay. We eat a variety of foods, and some are more prone to causing tooth decay than others.

Undiagnosed diabetics with uncontrolled high blood sugar will probably have higher rates of tooth decay.

Some teeth are less resistant to acids than other teeth. Teeth containing fluoride or tetracycline are more resistant to tooth decay. Also, John O. Grippo, D.D.S., has shown that teeth under mechanical stress will decay quicker when affected by acid. Its composition and the stress it withstands, as with braces, will make a tooth more susceptible to tooth decay.

The quantity and the composition of saliva affect remineralization. Anything that causes a dry mouth will decrease the saliva's ability to repair teeth. Medicines are usually the culprit. As they get older, people usually take medicines for their ailments, and these medicines cause dryness of the mouth. Tooth decay becomes a problem in older adults, especially octogenarians. Food has a definite role too. We should also avoid foods like raisins, dried fruit, granola bars, and even peanut butter because they stick to the teeth and make it difficult for the saliva to wash the sugar away.

We can fight tooth decay in a number of ways. We can use familiar mechanical means to remove foods that cause tooth decay, including brushing, flossing, toothpicks, and water picks. We can use mouthwashes that contain fluoride and attack plaque. Germicidal mouthwash with chlorhexidine gluconate also reduces bacteria in the mouth and fights tooth decay. Tooth-whitening agents also attack the bacteria that cause tooth decay. What we really need is a remineralizing rinse for patients with dry mouths. In the meantime, medicines that stimulate the saliva glands may be beneficial for patients with dry mouths.

14

Root Canal Treatment

What exactly is a root canal, and when do we need it?

When a dentist performs a root canal, he removes the soft tissue, or the pulp, inside the hard tooth. After the pulp is removed and the inside is cleaned, the hollow area left behind is filled in with a biocompatible material such as gutta-percha, titanium, silver, or silver amalgam. Although pure silver was used forty years ago, gutta-percha, a natural plastic-like material, is usually used today.

When are we certain a patient really needs a root canal? We're certain when the soft tissue inside the hard tooth is necrotic, or dead. Dentists see this on x-rays or clinically, but this tissue death may take up to six months to show up on an x-ray. However, symptoms may appear as swelling or a fistula.

Many times root canals are performed because of acute pain and not because of infection or death of the nerve. Balancing side guidance or group guidance could have been the cause of the pain. A patient with anterior guidance or canine guidance would be less likely to have a need for root canal treatment. Also, in such a patient, the root canal would be less likely to fail.

A tooth that needs a root canal will be painful when it's touched. It will also cause ear pain; temple pain, and pain while chewing, and it will most likely keep you up at night. Tylenol, Motrin, or aspirin generally will not make the pain go away completely if a root canal is needed.

Generally, in teeth that have more than one nerve, all the nerves die at the same time, but not always. This can cause an incorrect diagnosis, as can occlusion and sinusitis. Teeth with decay that need root canal treatment often fare better than cracked teeth that need root canal treatment because cracked teeth may be prone to more cracking. In the case of a cracked tooth, the dentist needs to find out what caused the crack in the first place. Was it occlusion, or did the patient bite too hard? Has the occlusion been changed after root canal treatment? Has the patient learned his lesson about biting too hard?

15

What You Can Do to Make Your Teeth Look Nice and Stay Healthy

There are a number of things you can do to keep your teeth healthy.

- Avoid smoking. Smoking is like adopting a systemic disease. It affects your whole body. Your gums will not be healthy; they will be prone to bleeding, and you will be more likely to suffer from osteoporosis. You are more likely to have periodontal disease. Smoking also stains your teeth and dries your mouth out, so you are more likely to get tooth decay. If you smoke, you will be more prone to infection. You can't have healthy gums, bones, and teeth when you smoke. The hot smoke is also likely to cause changes in the soft tissues inside the mouth.

- Avoid sudden, drastic changes in temperature. Teeth will crack when subjected to sudden changes in temperature. Drinking hot coffee followed by eating ice cream will cause vertical cracks in many teeth. Over time these cracks stain, and they will age your teeth.

- Avoid sucking on lemons and oranges or chewing vitamin C tablets. The acids will eat away at your teeth. Drinking soda can also damage your teeth, although I have very seldom seen teeth damaged by soda.

- Avoid biting your fingernails, pens, pencils, golf tees, etc. Don't open bottles with your teeth. Don't crack lobster shells with your teeth. Avoid eating hard bread and hard pizza crust. Many people break their teeth on hard pizza crust and hard bread.

- Don't drink coffee with a lot of sugar. If you put four sugars in a small cup of coffee and drink several cups of coffee a day, you're more likely to have tooth decay around your fillings and near the gum line.

- Avoid sucking on sugared mints. You're more likely to have a problem with tooth decay if you do this.

- Acid indigestion or gastroesophageal reflux disease (GERD) will damage your teeth. The acid will cause your back teeth to shrink. People who suffer from bulimia and patients who vomit a lot will also have this problem.

- Avoid anything that will cause your teeth to stain, such as blood, smoking, red wine, and ketchup.

- Make sure you have canine or anterior guidance. Go to a mirror and observe which teeth touch or make contact in excursions. If you don't have canine or anterior guidance, go see your dentist and have it corrected.

- Have crooked teeth fixed because they cast shadows that make other teeth look darker.

- Breathing with your mouth open at night may make your gums more red and puffy.

16

Biological Width, Calculus, Inflammation, Overhangs, and Margins

Every tooth and every dental implant has a biological width, which is the amount of soft tissue that has to cover bone. Bone should not be exposed in the oral cavity. The natural tooth or dental implant that comes out of the jawbone must have a ring of connective tissue so the bone is not exposed. The amount of this tissue must be at least two or three millimeters. A collar of tissue must separate the bone from the tooth or implant.

Dental calculus, a non-living, calcified plaque, can impinge on this biological width and cause the gums to recede slowly. Any pressure or insult to this biological width, such as slow-growing calculus, long fillings, or overextended crowns, will cause injury to this width. Injury to this width causes the bone to shrink. Once this bone is lost, it usually does not come back.

Calculus may or may not cause inflammation as it slowly creeps and impinges on this biological width. Very often inflammation is not seen next to calculus. Long fillings or crowns usually cause inflammation when they encroach on the biological width. This inflammation may last for a long time, and it will only go away when the bone resorbs.

Chronic inflammation under the pontic of a three-unit bridge may be present for many, many years, yet no soft tissue or bone resorbs because of this inflammation. A pontic is an artificial tooth that is mounted on a fixed or removal dental appliance and sits on the gum ridge. On a fixed bridge, the pontic is attached to two surrounding abutments, or dental crowns. When there is inflammation under a pontic, should this inflammation be classified as biological width inflammation or foreign body inflammation or pressure inflammation? Such inflammation is very common, and no one can explain yet why such inflammation does not cause bone or soft-tissue resorption.

Dead bone or reimplanted teeth become foreign bodies that the body wants to reject. Does calculus on a tooth also act like dead bone or a foreign body that the body wants to reject?

Sometimes when a tooth is extracted, the whole tooth can come out easily, but many times the bone around the root of the tooth may die, and then this bone exfoliates on its own. The blood supply to the bone probably becomes compromised during the extraction, maybe from trauma, causing the bone to die. The compromised bone dies and becomes a foreign object that the body then rejects.

Interestingly, I've seen a piece of glass come out of a patient's gum tissue years after the patient was involved in a car accident. This patient had complained of years of vague pain in the gum. Now I know why.

17

Tidbits

Keyes Technique In the 1960s, Paul Keyes discovered that streptococcus mutans in dental plaque was a transmissible infection that caused tooth decay. Later he advocated the first nonsurgical treatment for periodontal disease—cleansing of the teeth and gums by the dentist every two to four months; cleaning at home with baking soda, hydrogen peroxide, and salt; monitoring of the results by using a microscope to examine the bacterial debris found under the gums; and, if necessary, tetracycline therapy. I believe it's great to brush your teeth with salt to keep the populations of flora down, but does it really prevent bone loss if a patient is unhealthy or has bad guidance? Keyes was trying to make periodontal disease scientific. But did he?

Is it conceivable that we haven't isolated the right organism yet? Transplanting plaque, which contains a host of different organisms, will not produce periodontal disease. Because dental plaque causes tooth decay, and dental decay plaque is scientifically validated and follows Koch's postulates, it was logical to assume that dental plaque must also cause periodontal disease.

For many years, we thought that stress caused stomach ulcers, yet now we know it is not stress, but a bacterium called *Helicobacter pylori*, or *H. pylori*, that infects various areas of the stomach and duodenum. *H. Pylori* follows Koch's postulates in its connection with ulcers; stress does not.

Many researchers today feel that our appendix, a small pouch attached to our intestines that contains countless number of bacteria, is a place where good bacteria live. Is the plaque around our teeth similar to our appendix in providing a reservoir of good bacteria for us?

Tetracycline and Periostat Tetracycline is an old and versatile drug. But it does have side effects. It can cause yeast infections in women and prevent oral contraceptives from working. It can permanently stain adult teeth if given to children whose adult teeth are still developing. It should not be given to children under eight or nine years old.

But the tetracycline family of antibiotics can do some positive things as well. It can stop infections, which is why it's used to treat Lyme disease. Tetracyclines can prevent acne and stop inflammation. They are also used to treat rheumatoid arthritis.

If you find an old drug, with a new dose for a new disease, you can patent it and market it—so says the FDA. Periostat is that drug. Periostat is a low-dose doxycycline, one of the tetracyclines. Periostat works by reducing the activity of the enzymes that destroy tooth and gum tissue.

Matrix metalloproteinases are released in the inflammatory process. They are proteolytic enzymes—enzymes that break down tissues such as collagen. Collagen is also found in bone. Tetracyclines help prevent these enzymes from working. Low doses of doxycycline, as found in Periostat, have no antibacterial properties. Therefore, Periostat should not affect or change any flora. Periostat is marketed as a drug for the treatment of periodontal disease. Periostat, as prescribed, contains a twenty-milligram dose of doxycycline, while commercially available doxycycline is found in fifty—and hundred-milligram doses.

True incidences of bone loss, tooth loss, and periodontal disease How many people lose their teeth very quickly from periodontal disease? And what is the life expectancy of these people? Do the mechanical properties of the buildup of calculus cause bone loss? Should this type of bone loss also be called periodontal disease? The body compensates for bone loss, but this compensation can't be measured. Other forms of bone loss are confused with periodontal disease, so how do we clarify this issue precisely? If other major bacterial infections have been treated and been reduced by antibiotics, why hasn't periodontal disease been reduced similarly?

Are wisdom teeth like deep pockets? When should wisdom teeth be removed? Why don't most medical insurance programs pay for patients to have them removed? Thirty years ago, in contrast, nearly all the medical insurance companies paid for the procedure. Why do medical reference manuals now say it's generally unnecessary to have wisdom teeth removed? Who wrote these medical reference manuals in the first place? Who is right?

Erupted wisdom teeth very often cause balancing side function, and that's not good. It's important for dentists to look at a patient's occlusion, especially a patient with erupted wisdom teeth. Partially erupted wisdom teeth can cause local infection, a condition called pericoronitis. That happens when the gum tissue around the molar teeth becomes swollen and infected. Pericoronitis usually occurs when the wisdom teeth only partially erupt or break through the gum. This allows an opening for bacteria to enter around the tooth and cause an infection. In cases of pericoronitis, food or plaque may get caught underneath a flap of gum around the tooth. If the food or plaque remains there, it can irritate the gum and lead to pericoronitis. In severe cases, the swelling and infection may extend beyond the jaw to the cheeks and neck.

Are erupted wisdom teeth similar to deep pockets? Yes. Deep pockets are subject to local infections. Do these local infections usually cause bone loss? No, not usually. If they did, it would be easier to remove the wisdom teeth. The usual treatment for these local infections around wisdom teeth is debridement, gently washing the area with warm water, checking the occlusion, and antibiotics or extraction.

How often do these partially erupted wisdom teeth flare up? Once a year, once every five years, once in a lifetime? That depends on the patient.

Deep pockets around any teeth are more likely to develop acute, localized infections, and dentists use that fact as a rational for removing them. How often do deep pockets flare up? The usual time period depends on the patient.

Are deep pockets around teeth like the diverticula of diverticulitis? I think they are. Diverticula are small pouches in the colon that bulge outward through weak spots. If the pouch becomes infected or inflamed, this condition is called diverticulitis. Surgery is not usually performed on people with diverticulitis. The usual treatment is antibiotics.

When should fully impacted wisdom teeth be removed? That's not an easy question to answer. Dental insurance companies have minimum age requirements. And there are risks associated with the procedure, such as paresthesia, a long-lasting numbness resulting from nerve injury during tooth extraction.

18

The New England Journal of Medicine

On March 1, 2007, the *New England Journal of Medicine* published an article concerning dentistry, something it very seldom did. When such a rare event happens, every dentist takes notice. The authors of the article wanted to suggest a possible link between periodontitis, or periodontal disease, and cardiovascular disease by looking at endothelial function. The loss of proper endothelial function is a hallmark for vascular diseases. As an aside, it is worth noting that there are many studies of obstructive sleep apnea and endothelium function.

The authors conducted a study that divided a hundred and twenty patients with severe periodontitis into two groups, a control group and a treatment group.

The rationale for the study was that if inflammation in the mouth was reduced, reduced inflammation in the body would follow. The authors wanted to measure endothelium function, because cardiologists have studied it and feel it is a way to measure the cardiovascular effects of one's body. The brachial artery is what is they routinely looked at.

According to the results, periodontitis existed when there was probing depth of >six millimeters, more than 30% bone loss, and over 50% of a person's teeth were affected. However, since no one can diagnosis active periodontal disease, they had to infer that these patients had active periodontal disease. These were "well characterized" patients.

The authors excluded from the study patients with systemic diseases, including diabetes, cardiovascular disease, kidney disease, liver disease, lung disease, other acute or chronic infections, and patients who had used systemic antibiotics during the three months before the study began.

But why did they exclude those patients? Because they knew systemic disease and antibiotics could influence the periodontal condition? However, in the treatment group, they gave locally delivered antibiotic. Why? The control group had only supragingival scaling and polishing—cleaning above the gum. The treatment group had full-mouth debridement, subgingival scaling and root planing, teeth extracted and microspheres of minocycline, a type of tetracycline manufactured by Johnson & Johnson, delivered locally into pockets. Interestingly, Johnson & Johnson helped pay for this study.

None of the people in the control group had any teeth extracted, whereas the patients in the treatment group had an average of two teeth extracted.

The study lasted six months and examined a number of markers. The markers were looked at on day zero, day one, and day seven, and then at one month, two months, and six months. I don't know why they chose two months rather than three months. Traditionally, almost all patients who are treated for periodontal disease are monitored every three months.

Results of the study

The study produced a number of findings.

- Treatment reduced periodontal lesions—nothing surprising there.

- At two and six months, endothelium function as measured by flow-mediated dilation was better after treatment.

- There was little change in C-reactive protein, one measure of the level of inflammation present in a body, at six months. Interestingly enough, lowering inflammation in the mouth did not affect C-reactive protein.

I have many questions about this study and its results. I wonder how many patients were screened in order to select the participants. I also wonder what the true incidence of periodontal disease is in patients who don't have systemic diseases. Out of 1,079 consecutive patients who were referred to Eastman Dental Hospital for periodontal treatment over a year's time, 159 patients were invited to participate in the study. I'd like to know who usually gets referred to this hospital. How many patients were rejected because of systemic disease? How many were rejected because they didn't have enough disease? If they had excluded smokers, how many patients would they have invited? These are the important questions that need to be answered before we can determine exactly what validity the study's results have. How many of these 159 patients were healthy? If all 159 smoked, what does it say about smoking and bone loss?

The last paragraph of the article begins by saying that the severity of peridontitis seen in the patients in this study affects about.5% to 1.0% of the adult population in the United States. They had to eliminate almost 90% of the patients who had severe bone loss due to other factors. One therefore gets a more accurate idea of the number of healthy people who get the disease: one in every 1,000–2,000 people. If smokers are eliminated, that number might be one in every ten thousand.

The authors also reference this report on periodontal disease: Papapanou, P. N. *Periodontal Diseases: Epidemiology. Ann Periodontol* 1996; 1:1–36.

According to the abstract from Papapanou, "The interpretation of epidemiological data of periodontal disease is difficult, due to inconsistencies in the methodology used."

Dentists also have one more problem that we share with medical doctors, continuity of care. When different health care professionals follow a patient, information can get lost in transition. For example, if a patient is seen first by a nurse, then by a nurse practitioner, then by a medical assistant, then by a nurse's aide, and then finally by a doctor, how accurately do all these people report their findings on the patient's condition? Blood pressure and vital signs can be measured, but how a patient looks and feels are wide open to interpretation.

Dentistry is no different when it comes to measuring gum quality, oral hygiene, tooth mobility, and even tooth decay. All factors are open to interpretation. It is better when one person follows a patient than when the patient is seen at different times by different team members. But to be profitable, multiple players are needed. A team approach is advocated.

19

Summary

Most occlusal guidance problems are preventable or treatable. Over time, guidance problems will show up as bone loss, cracked teeth, painful teeth, headaches, decay, gum recession, abfraction, or TMJ problems. Unfortunately, the American Dental Association doesn't believe prevention is the best medicine for treating occlusal guidance. The American Dental Association believes that treatment is warranted only after problems develop, an alarming view.

Bone loss is confused with periodontal disease. There are many causes of bone loss. We do not know how much bone loss is caused by periodontal disease. Periodontal disease means different things to different people, but the nomenclature of periodontal disease is always changing. Periodontists want to implicate bacteria as the only cause of bone loss around teeth. This is well and good, but why doesn't their implication follow Koch's postulates? If bone loss is caused by bacteria, the condition must be transmissible and contagious, so how contagious is it? Should spouses kiss? We should see familiar patterns. We would learn a lot about the disease if we had good epidemiology. We need good diagnosis and staging. We could see clearer connections if we could establish that bone loss is more prevalent in patients who have certain other medical conditions, such as multiple sclerosis or abdominal aortic aneurysm, because we do know that periodontal disease is more prevalent in diabetics than in nondiabetics.

Because we lack good diagnosis and good epidemiology, dental treatment for periodontics and orthodontics is not as scientific as it should be.

20

Glossary

abfraction. The loss of tooth structure caused by tooth flexure or by biomechanical loading.

bruxism. The grinding of teeth.

buccal. Toward the cheeks, as opposed to the tongue.

calculus. Calcified dental plaque, also known as tartar.

endothelium. The thin layer of cells lining blood vessels. It is involved with many vascular diseases.

inflammation. A nonspecific immune response caused by injury, irritation, stimuli, or infection. Inflammation is not synonymous with infection. Inflammation may be chronic, acute, local, or systemic.

matrix metalloproteinases (MMPs). Enzymes that degrade proteins. MMPs are involved with many biological processes and with inflammation and wound healing.

occlusion. How the teeth touch when the jaws are brought together.

open bite. Space between upper and lower teeth when the jaws are closed; may be anterior or posterior.

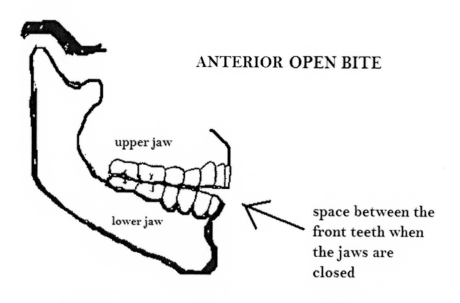

ANTERIOR OPEN BITE

upper jaw

lower jaw

space between the
front teeth when
the jaws are
closed

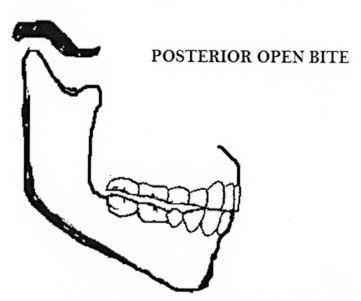

POSTERIOR OPEN BITE

**NOTICE THE SPACE BETWEEN THE BACK
TEETH WHEN THE JAWS ARE BROUGHT
TOGETHER**

osteoblast. A cell that makes bone.

osteoclast. A cell that removes bone tissue.

overhang. Excess amount of substance projecting from the tooth surface.

paresthesia. Numbness, usually long-lasting.

pathology. Diseased or injured condition.

plaque. A film of bacteria that builds up on teeth.

prematurities. Condition that occurs when one tooth touches first, before all the others, as the jaws come together.

retrude. Retraction, to force backward.

temporomandibular joint (TMJ). Joint that connects the lower jaw to the upper jaw.

21

References

Christensen, G. J. *Is occlusion becoming more confusing?* Jam. Dent. Ass. Vol. 135, no. 6, 767–770. 2004.

Dawson, P. E. *Evaluation, diagnosis, and treatment of occlusal problems.* St. Louis: CV Mosby. 1989.

Grippo, J. O. *Abfractions. A new classification of hard tissue lesions of teeth.* J. Esthetic Restorative Dentistry. 1991, 3, 14–19.

Lewis, R., and Dwyer-Joyce, R. S. *Wear of Human teeth: a tribological perspective.* Proceedings of the Institution of Mechanical Engineers, Part J: Journal of Engineering Tribology. 2005.1–18.

Newman, M. G., Takei, H. H., and Klokkevold, P. R. *Carranza's Clinical Periodontology, 10th edition.* St. Louis: Saunders Elsevier. 2006.

Randerath, W. J., Sanner, B. M., and Somers, V. K. *Sleep Apnea: Current Diagnosis and Treatment.* Switzerland: S. Karger AG. 2006, pages 151–159.

Schlossberg, A. *Dental Clinics of North America, Controversies in Dentistry.* Saunders. Jan. 1990.

Taubes, G. *Do we really know what make us healthy?* N.Y.Times Magazine. Sept 16, 2007.

Victor, L. D. *Obstructive Sleep Apnea.* American Family Physician. Nov. 15, 1999; 60 (8): 2279–86.

978-0-595-48083-8
0-595-48083-7

Printed in the United States
201677BV00003B/277-306/P